"Finally—A heart-healthy book full of realistic, commonsense ideas." —*Jacquie Craig, M.S., R.D., C.D.E.*

"This book is a wonderful, practical guide to a healthy heart. I highly recommend it!" —*Peggy Huddleston,*
Psychotherapist, author of Prepare for Surgery,
Heal Faster: A Guide of Mind-Body Techniques.

"An easy, fast, information-packed read that covers not only making the necessary changes for a healthy heart, but is a pertinent and interesting compilation of facts that can benefit the reader in a myriad of ways." —*Helen J. Ginsburg,*
author of From the Heart; Overcoming the Mental
and Physical Trauma of Open Heart Surgery
and spokesperson, American Heart Association of Colorado

"*The Healthy Heart Formula* is the best organized, most thorough treatment of the subject that I have come across. Your book allows anyone wishing to minimize their risk factors to get a complete review of the subject in one book. It will certainly fill a niche that has sadly been left empty for too many years. I wish I would have had access to such a book for my patients years ago." —*G. Scott Smith, M.D., F. A.C.C.*
Cardiologist

"*The Healthy Heart Formula* is a valuable addition for preventing, treating and even reversing coronary artery disease through appropriate dieting, stress management, and exercise. It provides the patient an opportunity to take charge and play a very active role in prevention and reversal of coronary artery disease, the number one killer." —*Mark V. Barrow, M.D., Ph.D.*
Gainesville Cardiology and Medical Center

The Healthy Heart Formula: The Powerful, New, Common-sense Approach to Preventing and Reversing Heart Disease. ©1997 by Frank Barry, MD.

Several recipes in this work appeared in a previous publication. ©1996 by Meadowbrook Press. Reprinted from *Eating Expectantly* by Bridget Swinney, MS, RD, with permission of its publisher, Meadowbrook Press, Deephaven, MN.

LIBRARY OF CONGRESS CATALOGING-IN-PUBLICATION DATA
Frank Barry, MD, with Bridget Swinney, MS, RD
The healthy heart formula. / Frank Barry, MD, with Bridget Swinney, MS, RD
        p.   cm.
Includes index
ISBN 1-56561-108-X; $14.95

Edited by: Jeff Braun
Cover Design: Terry Dugan Design
Text Design: David Enyeart
Art/Production Manager: Claire Lewis
Printed in the United States of America

Published by
Chronimed Publishing
P.O. Box 59032
Minneapolis, MN 55459-9686

The
Healthy
Heart
Formula

*The Powerful, New,
Commonsense Approach
to Preventing and
Reversing Heart Disease*

Frank Barry, MD

with
Bridget Swinney, MS, RD

**CHRONIMED
PUBLISHING**

ABOUT THE AUTHORS

FRANK BARRY, MD, practices family medicine and sports medicine in Colorado. Born in Jersey City, New Jersey, he moved to Colorado 15 years ago to take a residency in family medicine at the University of Colorado Health Sciences Center in Denver. He has always been interested in the whole person, not just their disease.

He received both his bachelor of science degree in psychology and his M.D. degree from Georgetown University. Disease prevention became an avocation after several years in practice. Family events also played a role. Sports medicine and exercise science helped in triathlons, century bike rides, and outdoor sports to which he aspires.

He lives the lifestyle he teaches at the Preventive Health Institute. His wife, a registered nurse with a master's degree in sports science, and their two girls frequently bike, camp, and play soccer together. Dr. Barry is the President of the El Paso County Medical Society. He lives and works in beautiful Colorado Springs, Colorado.

CONTRIBUTING AUTHOR BRIDGET SWINNEY is a registered dietitian with a master's degree in nutrition. She is author of *Eating Expectantly: A Practical and Tasty Guide to Prenatal Nutrition,*

which was chosen as one of the Ten Best Parenting Books of
1993 by *Child Magazine*. She works as a writer, speaker, and con-
sultant in Colorado Springs.

NOTICE

Consult your health care professional

Readers are advised to seek the guidance of a licensed physician or health care professional before making any changes
in prescribed health care regimens, as each individual case
or need may vary. This book is intended for informational
purposes only and is not for use as an alternative to appropriate medical care. While every effort has been made to
ensure that the information is the most current available,
new research findings, being released with increasing frequency, may invalidate some data.

ABOUT THE AUTHORS IV

ACKNOWLEDGMENTS XIII

FOREWORD XV

CHAPTER ONE 1

Twenty-First Century Medicine

The Proof that this Program will Work for You 1
Now, a Peek Into the Future..3
21st Century Medicine Today...4
Pleasurable Risk Reduction 5
The Proof..5

CHAPTER TWO 9

The Problem with Heart Disease

Introduction..10
Cardiovascular Disease States......................................13
Doctor, How Long will my Surgery Last? 15
Risk Factors..17
High Blood Pressure/Hypertension—The Silent Killer....21
Diabetes...22
Exercise 24
Smoking...26
Age..27
Family History 27
Stress 28
How Much to Change? 32

CHAPTER THREE   **33**

The Practical Way to Reverse Blocked Arteries

The Healthy Heart Formula 33
The Building Blocks of Food 35
Condiments 43
Off-the-Shelf Foods 43
Stress Management 43
Exercise—Move Your Body 48

CHAPTER FOUR   **51**

Eating Right, the Practical Guide

Ten Steps to Heart Healthy Eating 52
SAD (Standard American Diet) 57
American Heart Association Diet 58
Healthy Heart Formula Meal Plan 59
What Is a Ten Percent Meal Plan? 60
Planning Ahead for a Fat-Free Kitchen 63
Condiments—Spice It Up! 64
Herbs and Suggested Uses 65
Cutting the Salt 67
At the Table 70
Shortcuts to Vegetarian Eating 74
Recipe Make-Overs 77

CHAPTER FIVE   **81**

The Fat-Free Eater's Guide to the Grocery Store

Ten Ways to Shop Smart 81
Using the Food Label to Your Advantage 82
Healthy Foods Shopping List for Eating Right 90
Ingredient Guide to Vegetarian Eating 93

Storing Whole Foods 95
The Best Fat-Free and Low-Fat Foods 95
Questions You May Have About Fat-Free Food 97

CHAPTER SIX   99

Eating Away From Home

Fast Food...99
Good Choices 100
At the Salad Bar...104
Dining Out, Fat Free 105
Common Restaurant Foods that are
    Fat Free or Low Fat 108
Best Bets—Chain Restaurants 115
Healthy Food in Any Language....................................118

CHAPTER SEVEN   123

Women and Heart Disease—
The Weaker Sex?

Is There Sex Bias in the Treatment of Heart Disease? 125
Risk Factors...126

CHAPTER EIGHT   133

So What's Stopping You?

Stress, and How to Beat It!..133
Controlling Your Inner Self 138
Get on the Stick!..141
Seven Sure-Fire Ways to Improve Motivation! 142
Why Do We Fail to Achieve Goals?????? 145
Cheating..147

CHAPTER NINE   151

Move Your Body

Rate Your Fitness Level 152
It's Time to Set Up Your Exercise Program!!!.............153
Exercise Prescription 155
Monitoring Exercise Intensity 157
Cross Training..158
Exercise Equipment 162
Types of Equipment 163
Exercise for Fun and Profit..166
Warnings During Exercise..168
Fitness and Longevity..170

CHAPTER TEN   173

Kick the Habit

Stop Smoking Program...173
How Much Does Smoking Cost? 174
A Practical Program to Quit and Stay Quit 176
The Smoke Test—How Dependent Are You?.............177

CHAPTER ELEVEN   181

Should I Be Taking a Supplement?

Vitamins, Minerals, and Your Heart 181
Vitamins 182
Minerals 187

CHAPTER TWELVE   193

Pharmaceuticals

Drug Therapy 193
Factors in Drug Therapy 195

Waste and Duplication in the Industry *197*

What Will Companies Do to Sell the Product? *198*

CHAPTER THIRTEEN   **201**

A Word on Cancer Prevention

National Cancer Institute News *201*

The Case for Lifestyle and Cancer Prevention *202*

Case-by-Case Cancer Prevention *204*

CHAPTER FOURTEEN   **207**

Delightful, Delicious, Delectable Recipes

What You Will Find *207*

Breakfast Ideas *207*

Lunches On the Go *208*

Fifteen-Minute Meals *209*

A Month of Dinner Menus *212*

About the "Healthy Heart Formula" Recipes *216*

CHAPTER FIFTEEN   **283**

Choices

Postscript *286*

REFERENCES   **287**

SUGGESTED READINGS   **292**

INDEX   **297**

ACKNOWLEDGMENTS

As a first time author, I had no idea how difficult this project would turn out to be. I hope you, the reader, will gain from perusing this book.

I want to thank my family, Mary, Colleen, and Megan for putting up with my hours in front of the computer. Also to Bridget Swinney for help in the dietary arena, and as a valued contributor.

I owe a debt of gratitude to my friend and author Zoltan Malocsay, for the invaluable assistance he provided. Susan Hyne spent many hours editing and her suggestions were right on the mark. G. Scott Smith, cardiologist extraordinaire, has been supportive through the process and added his expertise to the revisions. I am eternally grateful.

The staff of the Preventive Health Institute, including Craig Engle, L.C.S.W., and Laurin McCrary, M.S., have lent their expertise and enthusiasm.

My extended family, including "Uncle Dave" Howes and Aunt Dorothy Zimmerman have taught me more on a practical level than words can say.

As a medical professional, I wish to pay homage to the giants in the field: the real pioneer, Nathan Pritikin, and to Kenneth Cooper, M.D.; John McDougall, M.D.; and Dean Ornish, M.D.

A private word to all my patients who taught me the practical aspects of their lives, and by doing so, brightened my life immeasurably. Thank you all for sharing such intimacy with your physician.

My only wish is that you could have known my father as I did. He was an exceptional man.

—*Frank Barry, M.D.*
Colorado Springs, Colorado

I wish to first thank my husband, Frank, and my sons, Nicolas and Robert, for their patience while I spent many hours at the computer and made many messes in the kitchen. And to my sisters, Judy and Colleen, my Dad, and Nicole for all their support.

I'd like to thank Frank Barry for getting me involved in the Preventive Health Institute—who would have known that it would lead to a book! Also, for giving my husband the knowledge he needed about heart disease to learn that he did have a choice.

I'd also like to thank all my friends and co-workers for their support, especially Wayne Valey, Kathy Glaaser, R.D., Kathy Fraser, Jacquie Craig, R.D., Ann Snyder, R.D., from the Gladstone Institute, and Mary Peet, R.D.

And for help in tasting products and testing recipes: Kathy Fraser, Julie Branscomb, Debbie Russell, Lori Hannah, R.D., Norma Robinson, R.D., Janet Boyd, Sheryl Stampher, R.D., Ceacy Thatcher, Nancy Oshner, Todd Rowader, R.N., Wendy Gregor, R.D., Dan Mayotte, Carol Williams, and Tina Fulton. Thanks to Ceacy Thatcher, Patty Magliato, Norma Robinson, R.D., and Shirley Lippincott, R.D., for the use of their recipes.

Thanks to my colleagues at Memorial Hospital and the Spring 1995 Behavior Modification Weight Loss Classes at Memorial Hospital for help in tasting fat-free products and recipes.

Special thanks go to Jeff Braun, our editor, who made the process painless; Claire Lewis and David Enyeart, for their production and design skills; and thanks to everyone at Chronimed Publishing for their support.

—*Bridget Swinney, M.S., R.D.*

FOREWORD

Preventive Health Institute

On the day of my college graduation I was awakened by a call from my parents' hotel. My father had just died of a sudden heart attack! He was only 53.

Stunned, devastated, I remember wondering if this is all that life is about: Work hard, get plenty of "standard medical care" and drop dead before you can see your child graduate. To lots of people, that's all there is. Millions die early, suddenly, needlessly. That was my introduction to heart disease, America's number one killer.

I went on to medical school at Georgetown, thinking that life should be better than what my father suffered—longer than that, richer, fuller, with time to enjoy family and accomplishments. But I was scared because a family history of heart disease is a major risk factor. Now the Grim Reaper had his finger at me, whispering, "Next?"

As it turned out, my aunt was next.

When my Aunt Dorothy had a heart attack, I was immersed in the usual medical training. Don't "blame" patients for their illness. Don't expect a measure of personal responsibility from people for their health. Drugs are the first line of defense. Surgery is the ultimate defense. If these don't work, write the patient off with the deadly dismissal "there's nothing else we can do."

But Aunt Dorothy wouldn't stand for that. She had been the picture of health! So when I learned that her cholesterol level was over 300, I was shocked. Then she started to have allergic reactions to all the cholesterol-lowering drugs, and I got frightened. What could I do to help? Immediately I thought of surgery, but she wanted to explore other possibilities. Yes, I had heard of Nathan Pritikin, but wasn't he a kook from California?

Dorothy's remarkable recovery from heart disease on a program of low-fat eating and exercise not only piqued my interest, it made me eternally thankful! At last, I saw something that worked!

I researched the work of Kenneth Cooper, M.D., inventor of the "aerobics" concept. His continuing work has been accepted and embraced by the sports medicine community, if not the heart disease community. My brother-in-law introduced me to the work of John McDougall, M.D., and the concept that disease could be cured by proper nutrition. Anne Frahm's *A Cancer Battle Plan* introduced me to the term "SAD," for Standard American Diet. Could all the favorite American foods like burgers, fries, and shakes that I had enjoyed my whole life be causing the diseases which plague modern Americans? The evidence was mounting.

As I continued my study of heart disease and prevention, I became interested in cholesterol and its metabolism. Imagine my surprise when, at a conference, I learned that an integrated approach of diet, exercise, and stress reduction advocated by Dean Ornish, M.D., had actually reversed heart disease! I considered this a world-class scientific achievement! No longer would doctors "plug the hole" in the proverbial dike. We could actually reverse the number one killer!

Nevertheless, the general medical community remains uncomfortable about implementing these advances. And there are no internationally known pharmaceutical companies willing to fund further research on the beneficial effects of a low-fat diet on heart disease and cancer. The standard medical protocols remain "usual and customary care." If Americans don't take control of their own care, then "usual and customary" is all they're going to get.

The Purpose of this Book

It was frustration—even desperation—that urged me to found the Preventive Health Institute. I wanted to put all these new tools to work!

The Preventive Health Institute is a team of professionals from the fields of exercise physiology, mental health, nutrition, and medicine who work together to teach people—victims of heart disease and hardening of the arteries—to take back control of their lives. Based in Colorado Springs, Colorado, away from academic medical centers, the Institute has been successful in helping ordinary people rather than "subjects" in a research program. This highly personal approach made us concentrate on down-to-earth interventions to change the health and lives of working people.

We have found out what other programs haven't: why most prevention/reversal programs fail. As it turns out, the answer is as clear as the nose on your face.

People go for the small, easy changes at first. When a small, hard-to-measure benefit occurs, most just give up with a "what's the use?" They don't feel better, they just feel deprived. "Wow, my cholesterol dropped 5 points—Big deal."

The secret: big changes, big benefits. All at once. After a week or two, when you don't need to look for benefits with a magnifying glass because you already feel them, you'll be happy. The improvements will keep you coming back for more.

So what follows is a truly practical program to prevent and reverse heart and vascular disease for those willing to make the changes. This program actually works to help those at most risk. By good fortune, it is an excellent information source for worried spouses and loved ones. Even more, the program demonstrates a lifestyle that can benefit everyone who is willing to make the change to a better life.

But I know what you're thinking; I know what you fear.

You don't want to live like a hamster, caged by your disease, forced to eat a hamster's diet and exercise endlessly on a hamster's treadmill, just to save your miserable life.

That's no life for a human being. I agree.

And that's why you've opened the right book! This is not a program of deprivation and hardship; this is a program of abundance and fun. Once you make the change, you can rid yourself of your disease and free yourself from its cage. At last, you'll find yourself in a world that is a grand buffet of delicious and exciting foods, an unfolding abundance of different eating pleasures. You can live a wonderful life with less stress and more fun! You can become more active, stronger, better able to enjoy each new day. With some practical help—and an open mind—you can literally eat, drink, and be merry, and live to enjoy your family and your accomplishments as my father never did.

Sound too good to be true? You'll earn the results, believe me! It'll take some doing, some work, some close attention, because this is applied science, not magic. But we call this a practical guide because you really can do it, and it really does work. If you make the change, you can be the living proof just like the others who've tried.

My prescription is: make the change using the Healthy Heart Formula!

CHAPTER ONE

TWENTY-FIRST
CENTURY MEDICINE

"To boldly go where no man has gone before"
—*Star Trek*

Read this chapter for:
+ Present Therapy of Heart Disease
+ 21st Century Advances, Available Today
+ Pleasurable Risk Reduction

The Proof that this Program will Work for You

Imagine Fred, your loved one, experiencing chest pains. His doctor thinks it's due to blockage of a heart artery. Fred is told to take medication (a beta blocker and nitroglycerine). Dutifully following advice, he finds he has headaches and feels tired as side effects. He can no longer take his daily walk because of fatigue, and he is not very happy!

When Fred returns to the doctor, a check on cholesterol shows it is rising. The chest discomfort, although better, is still present. He is referred to a cardiologist.

The cardiologist is a caring, cautious man. After reviewing the treadmill test results, which reveal several minor abnormalities, he recommends cardiac catheterization. The Operative Permit states, "I will cut a small hole in your artery, and push a catheter through it into your heart. Then, after injecting dye into the catheter, I will take a series of pictures. These will show any

2   blockage. Side effects are minimal, but include bleeding, infection, damage to the artery, and cardiac arrest."

The test is scheduled the next day. Although apprehensive, Fred sails through without complications. When reviewing the results, the cardiologist notes blockages of 75 percent in the right coronary artery, and 30 to 40 percent in the left anterior descending and left circumflex arteries. (These are the three largest, most important sources of nourishment to the heart.) In his conference with the patient, he dismisses the left artery blockages as "minimal." The right artery, however, must have immediate angioplasty to "avoid a heart attack." Now frightened, Fred agrees and has an angioplasty the next day. The balloon is blown up to 12 atmospheres of pressure, crushing the plaque, partially dilating the artery.

Six months later, on-and-off chest pain returns. Fred rushes to see the cardiologist, who orders immediate catheterization. The site of the angioplasty is, unfortunately, completely blocked. In addition, the left artery blockages look "ratty" or irregular. In conference with Fred, the cardiologist recommends immediate bypass surgery, and sends in the surgeon.

The surgeon, after agreeing with the cardiologist, says there is time in his schedule tomorrow. Otherwise, "you might have to wait till next week, and I don't know what might happen in the meantime."

Fred is feeling apprehensive and insecure about his future. He signs the permit, which states, "After putting you to sleep, we use a small saw to cut your sternum (breastbone). Your heart is then stopped. Your circulation is controlled by machine pump. Veins from your leg are used to bypass the blocked arteries. Your heart is then re-started. Possible side effects are infection, bleeding, pneumonia, heart attack, stroke, and death."

At surgery the next day, the surgeon finds a scar on the heart, indicative of a heart attack from the right artery blockage. He is able to bypass the right and both left arteries. Fred, feeling better save for his chest, is ready to go home.

On the day of hospital discharge, the surgeon says "the operation was a complete success. I was able to bypass the blockages. Except for the little scar I found, your heart is working well. Go home, be careful, eat right, exercise, reduce stress, and enjoy yourself. Any questions?"

As Fred opens his mouth to ask "but doctor, how long will my surgery last?" the surgeon is out the door. "See you in two weeks in the office. I have another emergency surgery to perform."

Fred leaves feeling perplexed. "Am I cured? Then why do I have to be careful? And just what does 'eat right' mean, anyhow? And how do I enjoy myself if I can't enjoy myself?" Fred's wife, Wilma, worries that Fred doesn't understand the meaning of this illness to their life and happiness.

Now, a Peek Into the Future...

Fred's granddaughter is watching a hologram from her dear, departed granddad:

> How fortunate you are, Sarah. From your early years in junior high school when you were 8, through college at age 14, you have been exposed to the concepts of 21st century medicine. And now you will be a doctor! I am very proud and also more than a little relieved.
>
> Today, heart disease and hardening of the arteries is not the problem it once was. Instead of waiting for disease to happen, doctors believe that "an ounce of prevention is worth a pound of cure." They teach everyone exactly how and why they can prevent the major killers. They have refined "pleasurable" risk reduction to a science. Let me tell you how things have changed since I had my heart attack.
>
> After meat advertising was banned, people realized they had many choices in food and other aspects of their lifestyle, and

4

felt less pressure to make bad health choices. And when these choices led not only to heart health, but less cancer and greater happiness, the movement grew. Research proved the power of good mental attitude. "Believing is seeing," (using the power of your will to make positive change—rather than seeing is believing) and positive attitude became powerful therapeutic tools of medicine. People like me finally figured out the meaning of our disease to our lives.

Now, of course, everyone exercises, even those with disease. We know exercise helps rather than hurts a damaged heart.

The pursuit of meaning in life, after setting clearly defined goals, became the "vaccine" of 2010. As more people were expected to take personal responsibility for their health, more actually did so. With the power of food to prevent disease, instead of cause it, and the vaccine of happiness, coupled with .education on good and bad choices, the world is a better place to live. Since women are now treated equally to men in medicine, in professional opportunity, and in the therapy of disease, you, Sarah, can practice the 21st century specialty, the specialty of practical proven prevention. Here's to your heart, your health, and your happiness. Prevent heart disease so your patients won't have to reverse it.

21st Century Medicine Today

The Preventive Health Institute practices 21st century medicine. I will present detailed descriptions of pleasurable, concise, and practical guidelines on food and its power to heal, stress reduction and its therapeutic effects, and exercise.

- ◆ All the people who come to the Preventive Health Institute have one thing in common. They have heart disease (hardening of the arteries). They have been helped by 21st century medicine.

- Those concerned with *preventing* heart disease or stroke can also benefit.
- Anyone planning for a healthy, long, happy retirement would be well advised to follow the Pleasurable Risk Reduction Plan. It lets you enjoy the fruit of your labor alongside your family.
- Get rid of side effects that make you feel ill.

Pleasurable Risk Reduction

The following are powerful predictors of future cardiac health. They also can help you "feel like" making the change:

- Happiness and lack of depression
- Marital satisfaction
- Higher education level
- Owning a pet
- Taking a nap or slowing down on the job
- Having one or two drinks of alcohol a day (only if you already drink!)
- Gentle, pleasurable physical activity most every day
- Based on a close look at the meaning of your life, make appropriate health-enhancing choices about your food, your job, your family, and your happiness

Make the change! Get rid of your disease.

From a concept by David S. Sobel (used with permission from Robert Ornstein and David Sobel: Healthy Pleasures. *New York: Addison-Wesley, 1989). (Reference 1)*

The Proof

I will briefly review the scientific studies showing the benefits of 21st century medicine in reversing heart disease. If you or your doctor have questions, look up the scientific references. It is very important to have a rational, reasonable plan before you embark on the changes outlined in this book. Convince yourself that this

6   plan will work for you. (See also suggested reading, page 292.)

DIET AND EXERCISE

◆ *Lifestyle Heart Trial.* Proves that people with hardening of the arteries can reverse the disease without medicine or surgery. Changes included a 10 percent low-fat vegetarian diet, smoking cessation, comprehensive stress management, and exercise. Of interest, the control group got worse. They stayed on the American Heart Association's Step 2 diet (27 percent fat). (Reference 2)

◆ *St. Thomas Atheroma Regression Study.* One arm of this study consisted of a 27 percent low-fat diet, weight loss to ideal body weight, and daily exercise. Regression of heart disease was seen in 38 percent of this group. Another part of this study used drugs and was also successful. (Reference 3)

◆ *Changes in Myocardial Perfusion...,* the five year follow-up to Dr. Ornish's initial Lifetyle study. Specialized scans of the heart (PET scans) were used to prove that low-fat diet, mild to moderate exercise, stress management, and group support do cause regression of heart artery blockages. Also, the function of the heart improves. (Reference 4)

DRUGS, DIET, AND EXERCISE

◆ *Coronary Drug Project.* Proved that nicotinic acid or niacin reduced recurrent heart attacks, 8.9 versus 12.2 percent after 6 years. Also, after 10 years, all-cause death was reduced, 58.2 versus 52 percent. (Reference 5)

◆ *Pravastatin Multinational Study Group for Cardiac Risk Patients.* Proved that pravastatin reduced the risk of serious cardiovascular events, 0.2 versus 2.4 percent, after 6 months. (Reference 6)

◆ *Familial Atherosclerosis Treatment Study.* Proved that two sets of drugs (lovastatin and colestipol, and niacin and colestipol), both lowered cholesterol and caused

regression (32 percent for lovastatin and 39 percent for
niacin groups). (Reference 7)

◆ *Cholesterol Lowering Atherosclerosis Study.* Proved that
after bypass surgery, a low-fat diet, colestipol, and niacin
caused regression in 18 percent after 4 years, versus 6.4
percent of controls. (Reference 8)

◆ *Scandinavian Simvastatin Survival Study.* Proved that a
cholesterol-lowering drug reduced, in 5.4 years, the overall
risk of death by 30 percent. Also decreased the risk of coronary death by 42 percent. All participants had previous
heart disease. (Reference 9) Expert physicians, comment-
ing on this study, feel it will enable doctors to treat heart
disease differently, with less surgery and angioplasty.

◆ *The "West of Scotland Study."* This is the first study to
prove, in those who have not yet suffered a heart attack
but have high cholesterol, that lowering the cholesterol
with pravastatin lowers the risk of heart attack and death.
Further, these 6,000 men were followed for almost 5 years
and were not adversely affected by this drug therapy,
proving the safety of cholesterol lowering drug therapy.
(Reference 10)

Greater benefits are gained from greater lowering of the LDL
cholesterol, the "bad" cholesterol. How low? It is Dr. William
Castelli's opinion (the director of the landmark Framingham
heart study), that an LDL cholesterol of 150 or less is protective
of heart attack in almost all circumstances!

The benefits of 21st century medicine overall consist of
reduction in chest pain, heart attack, and stroke (the benefits
even extend to decrease in cancer). Participants note an
enhanced quality of life. They also often find meaning for their
life and their disease. Even those without regression who were
successful in reducing LDL cholesterol benefited! The magni-
tude in some studies was 70 to 80 percent reduction in bad outcomes compared to the control group!

CHAPTER TWO

THE PROBLEM WITH HEART DISEASE

"Live sensibly—among 1,000 people, only one dies a natural death, the rest succumb to irrational modes of living."
—Maimonides, 12th century philosopher

This chapter reviews the medical aspects of hardening of the arteries. What it causes, such as:

◆ stroke and dementia
◆ claudication
◆ kidney failure
◆ heart attack, heart failure, angina
◆ a miserable, painful existence

The process of atherosclerosis revolves around "risk factors." Learn about:

◆ cholesterol
◆ hypertension/high blood pressure
◆ diabetes
◆ exercise
◆ smoking
◆ the effects of age, family history
◆ stress, the great killer

A buddy of mine, retired from the insurance business, told me what the problem with heart disease was. "I sold retirement plans for years. Save a little now, get back a lot when you need it. Money to travel, live on, enjoy the fruits of a life's work. But heart disease is like inflation. It cheapens every-thing. Now that I'm ready, it's worth less than when I started. I'm out of time. My heart is giving up on me!"

As she died that night in the Intensive Care Unit, husband at her side, all the retirement planning in the world didn't change her family's grief. For her, it didn't matter. Life was over.

Introduction

There is a difference between knowing and doing. Knowledge makes for interesting research and reading. However, when human lives are at stake, knowing is not enough. Every Tom, Dick, and Harry says you should exercise, eat right, and reduce stress. We will give you the tools you need to "just do it."

The practical aspects of our program are designed to enhance the doing. Research proves this program works in a way not possible with drugs or surgery. Now, take control of your heart, your health, and your happiness. And enjoy it!

This is 21st century medicine, available now. Many physicians think people are too dumb or too disinterested to learn how to help themselves. However, there is a large and growing movement of consumerism in the health field. People can and do make the decision to help themselves. When you do, know that

PRACTICAL POINTS TO PONDER

Signs of Reversing Heart Disease

You know you are starting to reverse heart disease when:
- *You feel better.*
- *You lose weight.*
- *Your cholesterol drops.*
- *Your physical endurance increases.*
- *Your chest pain diminishes, then vanishes.*

All it takes is the commitment to change!

the information in this book is scientifically based and proven to benefit.

Most of us today seek safety and control. Safety from crime, poverty, and disease. Control over our lives. Recent medical research has proven that heart disease can be prevented and even reversed! What does this mean? The hardening of the arteries which caused you to have angioplasty, or bypass surgery, or a heart attack can be opened up again. You can also learn the motivation to remain healthy in every way—physically, mentally, and emotionally. You can achieve both safety and control.

How can this program help you? It can improve your physical health. In addition, it can help you enjoy your life more fully, opening up new possibilities. Cancer prevention is a realistic goal. If these changes translate into longevity and vigor, so much the better. Even if they do not, the rest of your life can be lived to the fullest, enjoying all the pleasures life has to offer.

You may have spent your life feeling powerless about health and emotional well-being, trapped by inertia and depression, isolated from deep human contact. You may have given away your power. Others "learn" maladaptive behavior patterns which have outgrown their usefulness. Some feel unable to communicate, misunderstood. These behaviors can be changed. You can learn again the power to see and enjoy each day to the fullest. This leads to vastly increased productivity, creativity, energy, vigor, and satisfaction.

The knowledge conveyed in this program, coupled with a healthy dose of "believing is seeing," can lead to empowerment. Believe first, and it will happen. Wait to see it first, and it will never happen. The willpower and motivation to change come

FOOD FOR THOUGHT

You can gain the power of self-control. Lack of side effects. Freedom from the expense, pain, and loss of control of standard medical therapy. Proven results. 21st century medicine, available now. Make the change! Read the Formula!

from regaining control of your life. And once that step is accomplished, there is no limit to the positive benefits that take place.

Doctors used to believe that aging was inevitable. The more birthdays, the greater the inevitable decline in function: sexually, in daily vigor, and especially in heart strength. This is not true! Most of what we call "aging" is disuse (mental and physical), despair, and the ravages of an excessive lifestyle. That these factors can be reversed has now been medically proven (Reference 3). What we will convey, in a practical manner, is the *how* to accomplish your goal.

Your interest may lie in remaining "independent." For many, this means staying out of a nursing home, for others, traveling the world! Whatever it means to you, it may very well be your primary concern. You enhance your chance for an independent lifestyle with the knowledge gained in our program and this book.

One of my favorite people is Florence. She used to be sick. But something happened, inside her head. She decided to get well... and she did! Years ago, she embarked on her journey, did her own research. Exercise, eating right, improved attitude. She got rid of her problems instead of living with them.

Today, at 80, Florence has slowed down some. But she still takes her daily walk, and loves to regale me with stories. Although her old friends have passed away, she makes plenty of new ones. What a sharp mind. What a remarkable woman!

Please, help us help you. Start with an open mind. It's imperative to question, but leave a little skepticism behind. Try the "believing is seeing" attitude on for size. You may find that as you feel better, you will like the way it fits the new you.

Cardiovascular Disease States

I'll never forget an old veteran named Harry. A diabetic, he was one of my first patients at the Veterans Administration Hospital.

Harry was an engaging fellow, always smiling and ready with a joke. We got to see each other quite a few times during my medical training. Because of his diabetes and smoking, Harry had severe hardening of the arteries. This first affected his legs, and the pain of claudication (pain with activity, relief at rest) slowed him down.

But not his wit! It was always a pleasure to care for Harry. Through medical control of the diabetes, after angioplasty on the leg arteries, and during his aorto-femoral bypass surgery, the stories, the humor endured.

When the diabetes affected his vision, however, Harry seemed to fade. He was still pleasant, and always had a kind word for his doctors. But he was not the same.

The last year of his life was not a happy one for Harry. George, his son, was to graduate from high school. Angina, blindness, and recurring leg ulcers made life painful to bear. But Harry had a goal—to attend his son's graduation. When the heart attack came, we all thought he would never make it out of the hospital, much less to the graduation. Kidney failure, brought on by the fluid pills, made the situation worse.

The will to survive is strong. And Harry had a will. He pulled through, with a little help from kidney dialysis, and went home. Weakened, almost blind, he did survive to attend his son's graduation, and died soon after.

His son was kind enough to let me know that Harry appreciated all the care. It was bittersweet, feeling his kindness while seeing him suffer and deteriorate.

By far, the largest cause of preventable disease and death is cardiovascular disease. This includes clogging of the arteries all over the body. In the brain and neck (carotid artery), this can lead to stroke, memory loss, dementia, and loss of independence. This is termed "multi-infarct dementia."

In the legs, it causes claudication (pain with activity, relief at rest) and gangrene (death of the toes and feet). In the kidneys, failure leads to dialysis.

And in the heart, the clogging and eventual clotting can cause angina or chest pain, heart failure, heart attack (myocardial infarction), and even sudden death. These cause over a million deaths yearly. About half the people with heart attacks each year never make it to a hospital, never get the benefits of the "clot busting" drugs, but simply die suddenly. These deaths number over 450,000 yearly. Lumped together, this process of clogging and failure of the arteries is called atherosclerosis.

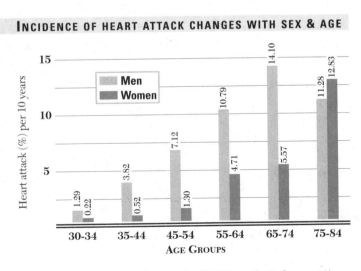

From the Framingham study of 5,127 people (Reference 11)

Doctor, How Long will my Surgery Last?

Therapy of atherosclerosis traditionally falls into two categories: medicines and surgery. Medicines give benefit to some, but the side effects may, and often do, outweigh the limited improvement (more on drugs in chapter 12).

Surgery falls into two types, angioplasty and coronary artery bypass grafting (CABG).

Angioplasty sounds great! Just push a balloon catheter through the artery until it crosses the blockage, blow it up, and blow the blockage away! Unfortunately, up to 50 percent of the blockages are back after only six months. In addition, the fracturing of the artery that occurs with each angioplasty can lead to bleeding and emergency surgery. Further, a clot often forms, causing the newly opened artery to have no blood flow due to the clot, rather than the atherosclerosis. Incredibly, research in the prestigious *New England Journal of Medicine (NEJM)* found that angioplasty may be overutilized by at least 50 percent! (Reference 12) That is, at least one out of every two procedures is unnecessary! Over 300,000 angioplasties a year are performed in the United States at a cost of $15,000 to $20,000 each. If, in the opinion of your cardiologist, you need a stent placed to keep the artery open, the costs multiply. And the biggest complication, even after stenting? Closure of the artery.

With angioplasty, experience makes a difference. A recent medical study proves there were fewer complications in the high volume hospitals and labs than in the lower volume situations. In fact, the authors propose increasing the minimum procedures per lab to 400 yearly (from 200 now). (Reference 13)

CABG surgery is equally popular. There is good evidence that enhanced survival occurs in selected groups (left main artery blockage, three vessel coronary artery disease, reduced left ventricle function, and two vessel coronary disease when the LAD artery is involved). (See the diagram on page 16.) However, most CABG surgery is done because of problems other than those listed above. Frequently, relief of chest pain is the goal. Research in the *New England Journal of Medicine* states that CABG is also overused one out of two times! It is performed about 260,000 times a year, at a cost of $40,000 to $50,000 a surgery. Seventy percent of vein grafts are occluded at 10 years! It caused heart attack in 8 percent as a direct result of the surgery! (Reference 12)

Cardiologists and vascular surgeons are debating which is the best method to use to "fix broken hearts." Isn't there a better way? Isn't it time to expand the debate to include natural lifestyle changes?

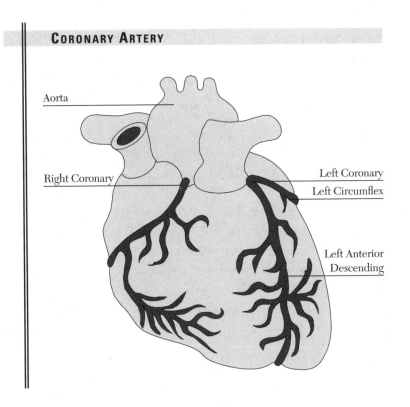

CORONARY ARTERY

Aorta

Right Coronary

Left Coronary

Left Circumflex

Left Anterior Descending

Risk Factors

If this section is too technical for your pleasure, turn to "Practical Points to Ponder," on page 31.

How is hardening of the arteries preventable and reversible? Doctors know that cardiovascular disease is caused by various risk factors. Reduce these and things improve. For you, improvement means less disease and disability, and prevention of early death. Change these risk factors thoroughly, and you can reverse damage already done. Let's get started.

CHOLESTEROL

I want to let you in on genetics. Many have given up the idea of changing their cholesterol levels. Stu was one of them. His father died at age 36. When Stu came to see me, he was 36 years old. It's true, he had a genetic form of high cholesterol. With a value of 350, he knew he had problems coming, but fast!

What he didn't realize is the power of 21st century medicine to reduce risk. We worked hard on a program of exercise, low-fat eating, and 40 milligrams a day of a powerful cholesterol drug called simvastatin. One month later, a much happier Stu found his cholesterol to be 225. Not perfect, but a heck of a lot better.

"I feel an early death, like my father's, is not inevitable now. I have a lot to live for, and now I see a way to enjoy life. The monkey is off my back!" Stu continues to lead a healthy life. He has even lowered his cholesterol below 200. And he doesn't fear death on a day-to-day basis anymore!

DIETARY FAT = CHOLESTEROL So when the label says "cholesterol free," watch out! The body needs building blocks for many tissues and chemical messengers called hormones. They are essential to the proper functioning of the body. The body manufactures all the cholesterol building blocks it needs every day. They are integrated into nerve tissue to speed nerve conduction. They are used in the adrenal gland and become chemical, blood-borne messengers to various tissues. They are even the building blocks for the sex hormones, which cause the secondary sexual characteristics (i.e., facial hair in men, and breast development in women).

When the body has too much fat in the diet (or because of rare genetic errors of metabolism of fat), it is not used in the normal way; it is changed into cholesterol. The cholesterol is transported through the bloodstream in large amounts, via proteins, to the tissues. Using the heart as an example, the bad cholesterol (LDL) "sticks" abnormally to cells in the artery wall. Over time, it is incorporated into foam cells which expand. These cause a small blockage in the artery wall (plaque), and the artery tries to dilate to compensate. Initially this compensation is successful, and blood flow continues unabated.

Eventually the artery cannot compensate (even before blood flow is obstructed). This is the most dangerous time for sudden death because the pressure on these cells can cause the plaque to "burst." This occurs when the artery is 40 to 60 percent blocked, but before blood flow is compromised. A big clot forms, suddenly shutting off the artery, causing "myocardial infarction," or death of a portion of the heart tissue. Over 90 percent of major myocardial infarcts (larger than 3 centimeters) are associated with plaque ulceration and rupture. (Reference 14)

However, it is also the time when the artery can fully recover its health and ability to dilate if the excess cholesterol is removed. The damage is not yet permanent! (This is the function of HDL, the "good cholesterol," mentioned later.) A low-fat diet (10 percent or fewer calories from fat) also removes excess cholesterol. This is known as the "threshold effect" and is known to occur well under the 30 percent fat level (recommended by the American Heart Association). Drugs, in high doses, can also remove plaque. There is some question whether they can restore ability to dilate.

When your doctor checks your blood, he or she gets a report on several parameters.

The total cholesterol can be tested on a random sample (i.e., non-fasting). It should be below 200. It consists of LDL cholesterol, HDL cholesterol, and triglycerides. The medical formula, for those of you who are interested, is:

Total Cholesterol = HDL + LDL + (Triglyceride ÷ 5)

Total cholesterol is not a very accurate or useful measure of risk, simply because it is made up of so many components.

LDL CHOLESTEROL is the "bad actor." This is the cholesterol made in the liver, in large amounts, and deposited in the arteries of the heart and other vital organs. The lower the level of LDL, the better. An acceptable level is 100.

There are several kinds of LDL. The worst is "oxidized LDL" which is denser and more atherogenic (causes more disease). We call this the "bad, bad cholesterol." Attempts to keep LDL in the less harmful form by using "antioxidants" like vitamin E have shown promise. Of course, keeping the body from forming any more LDL (by eating right) is a more successful strategy. There is some evidence that, in certain individuals, atherosclerosis can be reversed even without lowering LDL to 100.

HDL CHOLESTEROL is the "good" cholesterol. The higher the level, the better. The HDL transports the bad cholesterol from the artery wall to the liver where the body can remove it. Rarely, even when the LDL isn't high, a lack of HDL can contribute to heart disease (Reference 15). Aerobic exercise, weight loss, smoking cessation, estrogen replacement after the menopause, and perhaps an alcoholic drink a day can raise HDL. An acceptable level is 40, but the more, the better.

There is an interesting family in northern Italy. Because of a genetic mutation, their HDL cholesterol works exceedingly well. Despite their diet (they eat anything and everything they want!) they all live well into the ninth decade! If only we could all have this gene!

Some physicians report the ratio of total cholesterol to HDL. The ratio should be 4 or less. This can be useful to calculate risk of heart disease in asymptomatic people if the LDL is not too high and the HDL is not too low. For those with cardiovascular disease, the ratio is meaningless because they already have atherosclerosis. Their cholesterol is already too high for their own good.

TRIGLYCERIDES are another way the body transports fat through the bloodstream. Although not as directly harmful as LDL, in certain circumstances high triglycerides are a marker for accelerated heart disease. Diabetics can have high levels of triglycerides. At very high levels, pancreatitis (painful inflammation of the pancreas) can develop and can be recurrent.

To accurately measure triglycerides, the blood test must be done after a 12 hour fast. After eating, triglycerides rise rapidly as the intestines transport the fat in the meal to the liver. An acceptable level of triglycerides is 200 milligrams; desirable is less than 150. Often, high triglycerides and low HDL are found together. Triglyceride problems are helped by a low-fat, low-alcohol, low-simple sugar eating style.

If there is inadequate control of LDL over time, the deposits in the arteries continue to build. The artery can no longer compensate, and blood flow decreases. Although the body tries to form collateral blood vessels, frequently they are not adequate, and angina pectoris (chest pressure with exertion) develops. (Collateral blood vessels are new, smaller, parallel blood channels that can grow in number and size in response to stress.) Another factor causing angina is the inability of the artery to dilate. Angina might feel like "an elephant sitting on your chest" while walking.

A heart attack with blood clot may occur in the diseased artery. However, most heart attacks of a serious nature occur when the plaque, and the obstruction to blood flow, is relatively small. This used to be reported on angiogram tests as minimal or insignificant atherosclerosis. Why does this happen? The rapid and toxic buildup of the "bad, bad cholesterol" in the artery wall poisons its function. The wall weakens, and as soon as the blood touches these cracks in the wall, a blood clot forms. A crack might be caused by a cough, strain, or even the mental stress of balancing the checkbook!

Prevention revolves around decreasing LDL (and increasing HDL), by significantly reducing the fat in the diet, because FAT = CHOLESTEROL. The immediate benefits of a very low-fat diet on angina and heart attack risk are that the arteries dilate more easily and the blood can flow smoothly without slowing or clotting. This happens within two weeks!

One more thought on fat and cholesterol. Sooner or later you will have to decide if you want to live to eat, or if you want to eat to live. It is that type of choice with heart disease. If you decide you want to live, you will have to gather the people, places, and things around you that you live for, and count on them as a source of support. Make the choice wisely. Make the change!

High Blood Pressure/Hypertension—The Silent Killer

Hypertension, or high blood pressure, occurs when the arteries (outside of the heart arteries) constrict. This raises the pressure needed by the heart to pump blood. The causes of high blood pressure are many. Atherosclerosis can harden the arteries. Poor kidney function can cause hormone messages that raise the pressure (and the pressure can directly damage the kidney). There are many instances when doctors cannot find the cause.

Side effects of hypertension are deadly (thus, the name *silent killer*). It is the most important risk factor for stroke and is high on the list for heart attack, heart failure, and kidney failure. "But, I've always heard that blood pressure should rise with age," Aunt Gladys says. However, newer research has proven the higher the blood pressure, at any age, the higher the risk of complications (Reference 16).

Therapy begins with weight loss, exercise, and a low-salt eating plan. These have proven benefits. Stress and alcohol can cause hypertension to worsen and can be changed to help lower blood pressure. A low-salt diet may even help prevent osteoporosis. However, for whatever reason, these instructions are seldom followed even though they have no side effects.

Medical therapy consists of drugs, of which there are many. The several classes of drugs are: ACE inhibitors, which work in the kidney; calcium channel blockers, which primarily work on the blood vessels, but also in the heart; diuretics or water pills, which cause the kidneys to get rid of excess water; beta blockers, which slow the heart rate and dilate blood vessels; and alpha blockers. These all work to some degree. But they may have side effects which limit use. Recently, information on the deleterious side effect of calcium channel blockers has been reported by the news media (Reference 17).

The systolic blood pressure, the top number, is measured when the heart contracts. The diastolic blood pressure, or bottom number, is measured as the heart relaxes. An acceptable blood pressure is 110 to 120 (systolic) over 60 to 80 (diastolic). Even lower pressures can be normal as long as there is no associated weakness or dizziness. Try to keep your pressure on the lower end of the scale!

Diabetes

Diabetes mellitus is a common disorder of sugar metabolism. The childhood or early onset type is probably genetic or viral in origin and affects younger people. This type is rare and requires complicated, intensive insulin therapy. This should be managed intensively, as recent research proves that the lower the sugar measurements over time, the fewer complications.

The more common type is adult onset diabetes. Although

partially genetic, this usually is discovered in older people as they gain weight. Interestingly, with the proper amount of weight loss, 60 to 75 percent of adult type diabetes can be cured! Although both types share a high blood sugar level, the similarity ends there. The adult type is caused by insulin resistance and high insulin levels. Excess levels of body fat make adult type diabetes possible, and cause heart disease. (Reference 18)

Why all the fuss? Diabetes is a devastating disease, with many serious complications. Remember Harry from page 13? Diabetes is known to accelerate the atherosclerosis process. Also, many diabetics have a co-existing cholesterol (lipid) abnormality, which can be very resistant to therapy. There is a particularly serious combination of diabetes, hypertension, and high lipids which causes complications in the heart at a very high rate (Syndrome X). Diabetics also have a very high rate of vascular disease in the kidneys, legs, and eyes. This can cause gangrene and amputation in the legs, blindness, and kidney failure.

Therapy should begin with weight reduction. This can cure the disease. However, many people do not lose weight. Then, sugar lowering drugs are used. Unfortunately, although they lower the sugar, they frequently stimulate the appetite. The cycle then repeats itself, i.e., hunger, weight gain, higher sugar, and the need for ever increasing doses of drug. When the oral hypo-glycemic drugs (pills to lower blood sugar) no longer work, shots of insulin are used. Metformin (Glucophage), Acarbose, and other new drugs can be added. The same destructive cycle of hunger, weight gain, and increased dosage can occur. With the epidemic of "American diet" obesity, there are growing numbers of diabetics, all at potential risk of accelerated atherosclerosis causing vascular disease in various organs of the body.

A normal blood sugar is from 85 to 100, usually taken in the fasting state. Occasionally a glucose tolerance test is needed to confirm diabetes. This helps make the diagnosis of diabetes if the fasting sugar is normal.

Dan was adamant. "I'm not going to live with this! My father and grandfather died of diabetes. Help me!" With a blood sugar of over 300, sugar in the urine, high cholesterol, and fatigue, Dan needed some help.

Luckily, Dan was serious about not living with his diabetes. He had the common adult onset type. A recent weight gain of 30 pounds, combined with skipping his exercise program because of the job, brought out his diabetes. Dan sat down with his family and decided what was really important. The whole family decided to take daily walks. His wife supported his decision to get on a very low-fat eating plan.

When he returned in a month, Dan felt great! He was no longer fatigued. Even though his sugar was not yet normal, it had dropped by half. And he lost 15 pounds. On his two-month visit, at his ideal weight, his blood sugar was normal. As is common, as the sugar came down, so did the cholesterol. "All I really needed was to rethink my priorities. What good is it to make a little more, if I can't watch my kids grow up?"

Exercise

Television has the ability to greatly expand our lives. Most of us remember the day that John F. Kennedy was killed because most of us were watching television. Unfortunately, that habit is so ingrained that it has replaced exercise for most Americans.

Perhaps you are in the great majority of Americans. Does exercise consist of bending over to pick up the morning paper? This contributes to obesity, another American epidemic. Also, it contributes to physical decline and disuse (mistaken for aging in the past). In other words, if you don't use it, you lose it. This goes for heart function, breathing capacity, muscle strength, and mental capacity as well as sexual ability.

There used to be quite a debate about "fitness" versus "health," causing experts to advocate extreme methods of exercise (the marathon craze). However, recent research has proven that low levels of daily exercise reduce the risk of heart disease, stroke, obesity, and joint pain. These levels are the equivalent of walking most every day for 30 minutes. The *greatest* benefits of exercise occur when the otherwise inactive start *any* exercise, no matter how limited.

There are other benefits of exercise which the sedentary miss. After an exercise session, the appetite is suppressed for several hours. In addition, the metabolism (that favorite excuse of the overweight) is stimulated to a higher level. Often, people will comment on the satisfying mental relaxation that exercise brings. It is certainly a time which can be used for thought, reflection, planning, and rest of the mind. It decreases depression and stress. It makes insulin work more efficiently. Exercise is the most important factor to keep weight off once it is lost.

The benefits of exercise are not related to age. Recent studies in 80-year-olds have shown remarkable improvements in strength, endurance, and ability to concentrate. Exercise also helps to prevent falls, the precursor to hip fractures in the elderly.

Sedentary people have more hypertension, obesity, and diabetes. They "age" faster than their active counterparts. They often feel less productive and creative on the job. People who are more active have less fatigue, more energy, and they sleep better. Move your body!

Many people with pre-existing joint problems feel that it hurts too much to exercise, or it is too tiring. New advances such as water aerobics, water walking, and non-weight bearing machines (such as bikes) can allow people with these problems to become active and stay active. If you devote the time to exercise, you will notice the beneficial effects on mood, energy, vigor, weight, and endurance.

Many beginners complain of fatigue. This may be stress. Exercisers often note a lower stress level, which varies with the

26 duration of their program. Some people with heart disease fear that exercise will hurt them. The opposite is true! Exercise to enhance your longevity.

Read more on starting, and staying with, an exercise program in chapter 9.

Smoking

Nicotine is the single most addictive substance known to man. The nicotine in tobacco is more addictive than cocaine, alcohol, or heroin. No knowledgeable person will say that quitting is easy. But if you have heart disease you should not smoke!

Smoking kills more Americans than alcohol, AIDS, automobiles, and guns combined—every single year. Smoking causes accelerated atherosclerosis by a direct effect of the carbon monoxide on the lining cells of the arteries. Smoking also causes 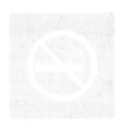 direct vasoconstriction (narrowing) of heart arteries, just like cocaine. It causes more sludging and clotting. It causes many types of cancer (see chapter 13, Cancer Prevention). Smoking causes bad breath, emphysema, chronic bronchitis, yellow fingernails, and old and wrinkled skin. Smoking kills the senses of smell and taste and robs you of the enjoyment of food and drink.

Has it been difficult to quit? Prepare several days in advance (see chapter 10 on preparing to quit). Your doctor can help with nicotine patches. You can chew gum, change your routine, cut down on caffeine (to lessen your nervousness and anxiety), and send your clothes to the dry cleaners. The worst of the withdrawal will be over in two weeks, but experienced abstainers know that the urge will last a lifetime. (It's like coveting thy neighbor's wife—it's what you do with the urge that counts.) Replace the habit with a new hobby, one that you can do 20, 30, or 40 times a day instead of lighting up. Do not smoke!

Stress may increase during withdrawal, but then it will plummet to new lows as you free yourself from the slavery of nicotine!

Yes, you may experience a transient weight gain. This lasts from 60 to 90 days, and can be lessened by exercise. Your health will improve, even if you gain a few pounds.

Learn more on kicking the habit in chapter 10.

Age

Age is an interesting risk factor. The more years you lead an excessive lifestyle with an overabundance of fat, food, and smoke, and a paucity of exercise, the more atherosclerosis you will have. Studies from the examination of childhood car accident victims have proven that fatty streaks in the aorta (the major blood vessel from the heart) begin by the age of 10 in Americans. Studies of wartime casualties have proven that atherosclerosis is well established by the age of 20. Studies of athletes have proven that the major cause of sudden death over the age of 35 is coronary artery disease! It is no wonder that, as we age, an increasing number of complications develop in the cardiovascular system, simply due to the passage of time and the work of risk factors.

Women past the menopause have accelerated atherosclerosis. The special problems of women will be addressed in chapter 7.

Family History

The medical history of heart disease in immediate family members can act as a marker for various problems, such as cholesterol disorders, possibly of a genetic nature. When the family has premature heart disease (under age 55), this is an additional risk factor. This deserves intense consideration because it raises your risk of having the same type of problem. You should help your doctor take a thorough, detailed medical family history. (Reference 19)

Stress

I love stories with a happy ending! I also see many people, like Claire, who start out miserable. We started out talking about smoking. She wanted to quit. It was soon evident that smoking was not the main problem.

"I'm cold. I can't relate to my husband or our friends. I just don't enjoy life like I used to!" Then the tears came. "I can't control anything in my life, my emotions, eating, sleeping, anything. I used to love life. Now I don't feel anything at all." As it turned out, these feelings had surfaced once before, just after high school graduation. But with a new job, new boyfriend, and a different outlook, the situation quickly resolved.

There were major problems among Claire's family. She and her husband hadn't had sex in months. He was working longer, and she didn't care. Their oldest child was acting up in school, and his grades were falling. His mouth was acting up at home, too. Claire just wanted to rest.

There were many instances of depression in Claire's relatives. Her father had been treated. He advised her to get some help. We discussed the situation for a long time. Because she was already feeling helpless, it took Claire a while to decide what to do. Finally, we agreed to arrange counseling and try an antidepressant.

This was a big step for Claire. But she was determined to break out of her "funk." And when she returned several weeks later, she did feel better. "Finally, I can sleep. I'm not great, but my mind behaves me now. When I feel sad, I cry, but I can feel happy, too. I can laugh again." It took three months, but she changed. Life had meaning. She sought new challenges in school. The love between Claire and her husband deepened. Quitting the nicotine habit went well. Her new job made her feel useful to herself and others. She told me how she appreciated the way she now functioned. "I never, ever want to feel depressed again!"

Our present day society is a killer! The pace of life has increased tenfold in only the last generation. All the innovations, inventions, and labor-saving devices have seemingly done the opposite—created less leisure time and more stress. Instead of peace and quiet, our faxes, cellular telephones, and pagers find us everywhere. Instead of limits to our work day, our work expands to fill 24 hours.

When the human race was in its infancy, we needed to be fleet of foot, strong, and determined. The hunter-gatherer life required quick reflexes and speed to run away from enemies or to catch prey. Over the centuries, humans developed the fight or flight response. Through a series of hormones (adrenaline and cortisone) transmitted through the bloodstream, our bodies received a quick burst of energy, our blood was shunted to only the most vital organs, and our senses were awakened. In the event of injury, these messages helped us stop bleeding and recuperate. In the event of a fight, the eyesight narrowed to focus on the aggressor, the strength increased, and the reflexes quickened. These responses helped the race to flourish.

Let's fast forward to the 20th century. Not many of us fight saber-toothed tigers anymore. The closest many come to a race may be to catch the morning bus. A confrontation may begin in the boardroom or the bedroom. However, physiology responds as it did in hunter-gatherer times: the elevated blood pressure,

FOOD FOR THOUGHT

- ◆ *Regain control of your life, health, and happiness.*
- ◆ *Be a willing, active participant in the change.*
- ◆ *Think about making all the changes at once. It's easier and more effective than the usual slow torture method.*

30   constricted arteries, and surge of adrenaline which now is not relieved by a fight or flight. The response is left for the body to dissipate while going about sedentary life—answering the phone, driving the car, and using the computer. Eventually this bodily over-response catches up, causing hypertension, coronary artery spasm, and maladaptive behaviors. We all know those who over-eat, over-drink, party excessively, take drugs, and smoke. These behaviors may temporarily mask the discomfort of stress but are certainly not the cure.

Do you feel isolated and alone, or lonely? We can fool our-selves that staring at the TV or taking a "Love Boat" cruise is social intercourse. However, real dialog on feelings and human emotions is lacking. Some people have simply never learned to effectively communicate and are left with platitudes (how about those Rockies!). Others, because of real or imagined slights, deliberately cut themselves off to avoid more pain. Still others lock themselves into a rigid pattern learned during a crisis. Many Americans are "disconnected" from the social structure of home, family, work, and neighborhood.

Modern Americans live in fear: fear of violence, fear of inti-macy, and fear of themselves. The pioneer spirit of adventure, that each day gave a new opportunity, is replaced by the drudgery of routine, joyless chores, tasks to be completed before retiring from life to the world of TV. This is the "Twentieth Century Malaise."

Doctors and psychiatrists call these states depression, anxiety, and despair. Also loneliness, drug abuse, and alcoholism. Drugs are often prescribed. However, with sensitivity, communication, and understanding, control of the body, mind, and emotions can be regained. This leads to enhanced happiness and well-being. Help close the door on maladaptive behaviors, and open the door to greater health of the body and the mind! When happi-ness and inner peace lead to empowerment and motivation, great changes are possible.

Others have risen above their foibles, and so can you. Witness the great works in art and literature of people, ordinary people, rising above despair. Use your peers, in a supportive group environment, to do the same.

Please ask your doctor specific questions you may have about your risk factors. They are very important in the quest to prevent heart disease. Knowledge is power, and this knowledge will help you regain power and control over your life.

The old saying, "an ounce of prevention is worth a pound of cure" is true. Those of you scared because of symptoms, your family history, or a long list of risk factors can benefit from this program. You will also realize a decreased risk of cancer of various causes. Some modifications are possible in those not yet sick, and I will point them out.

This program is designed for those with proven heart disease. Consider how serious another heart attack would be. If nothing changes in *your* lifestyle, nothing will change in your disease, or in your health.

The program can easily be adapted by those at risk of disease, or by those wishing to support their loved ones who are already battling for their lives.

PRACTICAL POINTS TO PONDER

Heart Disease Risk Factors

Hardening of the arteries is an epidemic! Risk factors cause it. Which of the causes of heart disease do you have the power to change?
- *High cholesterol*
- *High blood pressure*
- *Diabetes, especially the overweight type*
- *Lack of exercise*
- *Smoking*
- *Age or years with an unhealthy lifestyle*
- *Family history or genetics (change your "jeans"!!)*
- *Stress!!!!!!!!*

How Much to Change?

You may take the attitude that a little, gradual change at a time is easier than an all out, all at once revolution. Experience teaches that most people, after a little change, will quickly go back to the original behavior. This could be disastrous! Our advice, during this program, is to decide to change at once, and participate in an ongoing group support system. You've thought about it. You've prepared for it. Now, just do it! In this way, the change in taste of food, the slimmer waist from exercise, and the mental doubts are all combined with the improved physical well-being gained in the first two weeks. Eventually you will have to go all the way; show a sense of commitment and start from the very beginning! (More on change in chapter 8, page 146)

Make the change with the Healthy Heart Formula!

CHAPTER THREE

THE PRACTICAL WAY TO REVERSE BLOCKED ARTERIES

*"What you should put first in all the practice of your art is
how to make the patient well; and if he can be made well in
many ways, one should choose the least troublesome."*
—Hippocrates

The Healthy Heart Formula

OK. This is it. What to do to reverse heart disease. The plan consists of several cornerstones:

- Tasty, easily prepared low-fat diet;
- Daily exercise;
- Stop smoking;
- Stress reduction and the will to change;
- Self-awareness and group support.

They are all important, and help you in different ways. The following is a brief summary of the various components of the plan. With relaxation, stress reduction, and the will to change, you will accomplish great things!

QUESTIONS ABOUT THE HEALTHY HEART EATING PLAN

1. WON'T I TIRE EASILY IF I DON'T EAT FAT? The best source of energy is from carbohydrates, not fat. Excess fat in food turns to the fat you wear (around the waist). Eat carbohydrates to regain energy.

2. I'VE HEARD YOU CAN'T GET COMPLETE PROTEIN UNLESS YOU EAT MEAT. There are certain amino acids, the building blocks of proteins, that may not be present at each meal. It was previously thought that you had to combine complementary proteins at the same meal to have complete protein. (Beans and rice, for example.) However, as long as you eat a variety of foods throughout the day, you will have the correct amount and type of the necessary amino acids.

3. MY DOCTOR TOLD ME VEGETARIANS DON'T GET ENOUGH VITAMIN B_{12}. After about three years, our stores of B_{12} can run down on a vegetarian eating plan. If you don't have a reliable source of B_{12} from fortified foods or skim dairy products, take a B_{12} pill once a month.

4. CAN'T A LOW-FAT DIET BE UNHEALTHY? A diet can be unhealthy at any fat level—it depends on your food choices! Most would agree that it's a high fat diet that brings on most health problems. By following the Healthy Heart Formula Meal Plan on page 59 you can be assured a high quality plan for overall good health.

5. HOW WILL I KEEP FROM GETTING HUNGRY IF I DON'T HAVE A CHEESEBURGER FOR LUNCH? You may indeed have to eat more and more often on a low-fat meal plan. Low-fat foods pass quickly from the stomach. An interesting side effect is the absence of heartburn with a low-fat meal.

6. ISN'T THIS JUST FOR KOOKS? Examinations of eating styles of people who eat a lot of meat show high levels of heart disease, cancer, and contaminants such as antibiotics, hormones, and bacteria. True, media advertising pushes the average American to eat beef, chicken, and dairy. Media moguls may not be thinking of your health, however. They spend $60 billion a year to advertise their products to you and your kids.

7. HOW WILL I GET ENOUGH PROTEIN ON A MEATLESS PLAN? It is surprisingly easy to meet the Recommended Daily Allowance (RDA) for protein, even on a meatless meal plan. Many meat eaters eat about twice as much protein as they really need—which causes its own problems. The bottom line is—if you're eating enough calories, you're probably eating enough protein.

8. SO, WHAT WILL REVERSE HEART DISEASE? Research proves that a 10 percent fat eating plan for most men and up to 15 percent fat for women reverses heart disease in a comprehensive program such as ours.

The typical American eats far too much fat for good health (because Fat = Cholesterol). Protein in overabundance can cause physical problems. Carbohydrates, the energy food, have been given short shrift. Typical percentages of these foods, in terms of calories: fat 40 to 50 percent, protein 30 to 40 percent, and carbohydrates 10 to 30 percent. Typical "diets" make you hungry, and sometimes put the body into starvation mode, making it hard to burn calories efficiently.

On your new eating plan, fat = 10 percent or less, protein = 20 percent , and carbohydrates = 70 percent or more of calories. Why? It is medically proven that a 5 to 10 percent fat diet can and does reverse atherosclerosis. The "threshold for reversal" is reached. It is also proven that a 30 percent American Heart Association diet does not improve or reverse atherosclerosis (Reference 20). Few studies have been done to test fat levels between 10 and 30 percent (but people have unique thresholds for reversal). One thing you should not feel is hungry. When fat is eliminated, it opens up the possibility of more volume of healthy food. Your stomach and taste buds will not lack stimulation.

The Building Blocks of Food

For recipes, see chapter 14.

FAT contains 9 calories per gram, which is very calorie intense. Also, dietary fat is efficiently stored in the body, as "cellulite" or "love handles." There are different kinds of fat; however, all have undesirable effects, and all are unhealthy in excess. "You are what you eat" pertains to fat and your love handles!

Monounsaturated fat (found in olive oil or canola oil) has been called "good fat" although it is 14 percent saturated fat. (It is important to distinguish chemical compounds such as monounsaturated fats from foods such as olive oil. All natural foods which contain fat have some saturated fat.) There is no one "perfect food." See below for breakdown on different oils.

COMPARISON OF FATS			
FAT	%SAT	%POLY	%MONO
Canola oil	6	32	62
Safflower oil	10	77	13
Sunflower oil	11	69	20
Corn oil	13	62	25
Olive oil	14	9	77
Soybean oil	15	61	24
Peanut oil	18	33	49
Chicken fat	31	22	47
Lard	41	12	47
Beef fat	52	4	44
Palm kernel oil	81	2	11
Coconut oil	92	2	6

Source: U.S. Department of Agriculture.

Note: The sum of fatty acids may not equal 100% because some fats contain other components.

Polyunsaturated fat (safflower and corn oil) comes from vegetable sources. Again, foods such as safflower and corn oil also have some saturated fat.

Saturated fat is the undisputed worst for health. It is directly linked to production of LDL, the "bad cholesterol." Saturated fat comes mostly from animal sources, but is found in high amounts in coconut and palm oils and chocolate.

Synthetic fat is chemically treated, turning it into "trans" fatty acids which have a long shelf life, but correspondingly shorten your life. These are frequently listed on labels as "partially hydro-genated vegetable oils," often found in margarine and shortening.

Research in the *Journal of the National Cancer Institute* proves that men on a high-fat diet suffer an increased risk of prostate cancer (Reference 21). Women suffer higher rates of breast cancer (Reference 22). Both sexes have more colon cancer with the high-fat American style diet. (see chapter 13)

How many grams of fat do we need each day? Probably only 5 grams (2 percent of calories) daily to meet our nutritional requirements. How many calories in a pound of fat? We need to burn about 3,500 calories to lose a pound of pure fat. This equates to 10 to 14 days of walking 30 minutes at a good pace. How many grams of fat do typical Americans eat each day? About 100 grams—20 times more than the minimum!

Most of the fat in American food comes from four main sources: animal muscle (meat, chicken, and fish); dairy products (milk, cheese, ice cream); baked goods (pies, cakes, cookies); and condiments (gravy, salad dressing, sour cream). These are dis-couraged on your new meal plan. The other sources of fat are mostly from vegetable sources, such as nuts, avocados, soybeans, and tofu. Synthetic fats, usually found in off-the-shelf baked goods, are not healthy.

The minimal amount of fat ingested on the new meal plan will ensure the fastest reversal of atherosclerosis possible. Improvement can start in two weeks! For those with established heart disease, this is also the safest course to follow. For those with pre-existing heart disease, no amount of saturated fat is safe to eat.

I'd like to illustrate what a very low-fat intake can do. A general surgeon, Dr. Stanley Dudrick, put patients, deathly ill with angina and coronary blockages, on a "water" diet. Then, through an IV, he "fed" them a solution of amino acids (which are the building blocks of protein) and sugar for 90 days. The angina disappeared, blood flow increased, the patients got out of their wheelchairs and began to lead a normal life (Reference 23).

When they started to eat solid foods again the blockage rapidly returned because they hadn't learned to limit the fat in their diet. I know, this approach sounds drastic, but it is an example of proven, rapid results by getting rid of fat.

PROTEIN is necessary in small amounts for the structure of all the major organs, including muscle. Many trendy diets can produce a rapid weight loss, caused by loss of water and protein. This results in loss of muscle and subsequent weakness. Any weight loss originating from your low-fat meal plan will not result in these undesirable consequences.

Protein is made up of amino acids, nine of which are considered "essential" (they need to be consumed in food). The other amino acids can be made in the body, from the basic building blocks, and used as needed to build tissue.

Another source of controversy is the overabundance of protein in the typical American diet. Researchers have implicated loss of protein byproducts through the urine, linked with loss of calcium, as one cause of osteoporosis (the epidemic disease of

PRACTICAL POINTS TO PONDER

Food Tips

◆ *There is no one "perfect food"*

◆ *Moderation is relative, says Lynn Fischer, author of* The Low Cholesterol Gourmet. *"A guy has half a baked potato with sour cream. He eats half of his asparagus with hollandaise. He eats half of his raspberry pie with ice cream. And he eats half of his steak. He's hungry and he's had 1,000 grams of saturated fat and 1,000 milligrams of cholesterol." (Reference 24)*

◆ *One day a month, give yourself permission to eat anything and everything you desire. This reduces the daily urge to "cheat."*

◆ *A 10 percent fat eating plan can reverse your heart disease!*

older women which leaches the strength from bones, causing the "dowager hump" and hip fractures). The type of protein (animal versus soy) also seems to affect calcium balance. (Reference 25)

The average man needs only about 50 grams of protein a day; women about 44 grams a day. (RDA's are higher than average needs. However, recent research shows that some older people may need more protein than the RDA (Reference 26). One cup of navy beans has 15 grams of protein, 1 cup noodles 7 grams, and 1 cup skim milk has 9 grams with virtually no fat. Compare this to 3 1/2 ounces of lean ground beef which has 24 grams of protein, plus 18 grams of fat. The added bonus of protein—only 4 calories per gram.

PROTEIN IN FOODS	
FOOD ITEM	GRAMS OF PROTEIN
Tofu, 1/2 cup raw firm	20
Lentils, 1 cup cooked	18
Pinto beans, 1 cup	14
Soybeans, 1/2 cup	14
Quinoa, 1/2 cup cooked	11
Yogurt, vanilla nonfat, 1 cup	10
Split pea soup; 1 cup	9
Skim milk, 1 cup	8
Soy milk, 1 cup	7
Most grains and vegetables, 1 serving	2-3

CARBOHYDRATES are the energy food. Carbos are very efficiently converted to energy in muscle, causing increased muscular endurance. They contain only 4 calories per gram, allowing you to partake often.

Carbos come in many forms. Simple carbos (one molecule) are sugar. They are also called "empty calories" because they don't contain other nutrients, such as vitamins and minerals. (On the other hand, they don't have any fat either.) Many foods taste sweet because of added sugar, a good example being breakfast cereal. Those of you who count calories, beware of simple sugar for two reasons: the calorie count goes up, and our dental colleagues tell us they cause cavities. In some sensitive individuals, and especially in diabetics, too many simple sugars can cause a rise in triglycerides.

Complex carbos are known as starches. Complex carbos are absorbed slowly and are better for the metabolism. They tend to even out the blood sugar, protecting us from wide swings which would mean hyperglycemia, then hypoglycemia. Those with triglyceride problems do better with complex rather than simple carbos. When muscles are fatigued, complex carbos in the form of "sports drinks" (weak solution of complex carbos) are the most efficient replenishment. Additionally, complex carbos affect the metabolism, causing food to be burned off efficiently as energy, and not stored as fat. (Carbos have a high specific dynamic action. This means that carbos are used quickly and the process costs the body energy to do this.)

Fiber is a long chain of sugars, so long the body doesn't have enzymes to break it up. They are passed, unchanged, in the feces. They do attract water into the colon, speeding up the movement of food products through the colon and relieving constipation. This cures many rectal problems, such as hemorrhoids and rectal itch.

The greatest benefit of fiber, however, is the prevention of colon cancer. In countries where the colon cancer rate is low, the diet contains over 30 grams of fiber a day. Americans, with an average fiber intake of about 5 to 10 grams a day, have a much higher rate of colon cancer. Your new meal plan should have 30 grams of fiber. For the first weeks, this may take some adjustment: some people experience gas or bloating initially on a high fiber diet. This will not harm you, but colon cancer can harm and even kill you. Read more on cancer prevention in chapter 13.

Fiber prevents diverticulosis, inhibits polyp formation, and relieves constipation. It also makes bowel movements easy to pass, eliminating straining. See the list of high fiber foods on page 203.

Please also see the chapter 4 list of healthy foods which improve diabetes, lower blood pressure, and help you attain your optimal weight. These foods have a positive health benefit. Fatty foods, as you now know, have a negative health benefit.

Vitamins are important chemical compounds which help the metabolic activity of the body. They are required, in certain amounts, for health. The fat soluble vitamins, which are stored by the body, are A, D, E, and K. They are available in a healthy meal plan such as you are starting.

ANTIOXIDANTS: Beta carotene (which is converted to vitamin A by the body) is an antioxidant. Foods with large amounts of beta carotene include carrots, sweet potatoes, spinach, broccoli, cantaloupe, apricots, and asparagus. Eat these and you won't have to worry about a supplement.

Vitamin E is also an antioxidant. In doses up to 400 IU daily, it has been proven to have a beneficial effect on heart disease, probably by delaying or aborting the oxidation of LDL. In the dose needed to prevent heart disease, this may be the only vitamin you should supplement. Scientists gave over 2,000 people with heart disease a daily vitamin E supplement (either 400 or 800 milligrams daily). There was a 23 percent reduction in heart attack! (Reference 27)

Vitamin C is another antioxidant, readily available in fruitsand vegetables. It has been proven to have an anti-cancer effect. A dose of 1,000 to 2,000 milligrams a day is sufficient.

There is a comprehensive discussion of vitamins and minerals in chapter 11.

MINERALS AND OTHER NUTRIENTS: Minerals are essential to the proper functioning of the body. They are non-organic substances that aid the chemical reactions of the body in different ways.

Calcium is essential, not only to the bones and teeth, but also for the regulation of blood flow in the arteries. It is found in green, leafy vegetables, legumes, nuts, whole grains, and dairy products. There is quite a controversy surrounding the calcium in dairy foods. Because of the large amounts of milk and animal protein in our diets, the kidneys may excrete more calcium than is taken in (Reference 28 and reference 29). Therefore, a healthy protein diet, like we recommend, will help you achieve optimum calcium balance. Calcium pills are available, but absorption of calcium is higher in food than pills, so it is best to get your calcium from nonfat sources like high calcium vegetables or nonfat dairy products. See page 128 for information about calcium and osteoporosis and page 129 for food sources of calcium.

Sodium and chloride combine to make salt, as in table salt. They are essential to the proper functioning of the nerves, to fluid balance, and to acid-base balance. The typical American diet has 50 to 100 times the salt needed. Too much salt can lead to hypertension, edema, or swelling, as well as osteoporosis.

Iron is used in the hemoglobin molecule in the red blood cell. This carries oxygen around the body. Too much iron, especially in men, has been implicated in heart disease. Women seem to suffer less than men from heart disease caused by iron overload.

There are many other nutrients, all available on your new meal plan, which are not only essential, but serve to protect against various cancers. The typical American diet may sometimes be deficient in these nutrients because of lack of variety, a low fruit and vegetable intake, and over-processing. These substances, called phytochemicals, can protect against cancer. They are found in cabbage, broccoli, brussels sprouts, cauliflower, greens, horseradish, garlic, soybeans and more. Some phytochemicals, which are undiscovered, may be present in food, but absent from pills. It seems prudent to eat right.

A word about water. Water flushes the body of chemicals, helping to insure good kidney function. In combination with fiber, it helps form soft, easy-to-pass bowel movements. It can even help edema (swelling) by allowing the kidney to excrete excess sodium. Water can act as a natural appetite suppressant (if you desire), when taken cold and just prior to meals. Water can also act as a substitute for more harmful drinks, such as those containing too much caffeine (or other stimulants) or too much alcohol (or other depressants).

I'll answer your questions about supplements in detail in chapter 11.

Condiments

Lest you think your food will not stimulate your taste buds, be sure to have lots of condiments on hand. Some suggestions:

- ◆ No-salt seasonings, barbecue sauce (low sodium, oil free), fruit jams (pure fruit, no sugar), maple syrup, Dijon mustard, fat-free salad dressing, salsa (low sodium, oil free), Tabasco sauce, ketchup, and Worcestershire sauce.
- ◆ Most herbs and spices can be added to taste. Also, don't forget lemon juice, honey, vinegar, and various fresh and dried fruits.
- ◆ Many spices lose their flavor after a year. Be sure to keep your spices and other flavorings up to date, to appreciate the true flavor of your cuisine!

I'll help you set up your kitchen in chapter 5.

Off-the-Shelf Foods

For those not used to cooking at home, many new low-fat and no-fat choices are now available. See chapter 4, chapter 5, and chapter 6 for all the details.

Stress Management

Stress! You may live with it on a daily basis. Some people have a very visible reaction to stress such as wringing hands and pacing. They proclaim loudly, "I'm stressed out!" You, however, may internalize stress. Outwardly calm, you seethe on the inside.

Chest pain, headaches, diarrhea and belly pain cause no change in your demeanor. Why is this?

Stress consists of so many different factors. A typical high stress group consists of elderly white males. Research shows they have three times more likelihood of committing suicide than non-white males and six times more incidence of committing suicide than females.

In many societies, the elders are revered, sought after for their wisdom. Not so in America. Here, nursing homes and retirement communities are a growth industry. Social isolation is an American epidemic with many causes: fear of crime, television addiction, poor communication skills, and unwillingness to change.

There are several habits which can end social isolation. The classic method is to not be alone: get a pet, join a club, volunteer time in the hospital nursery or pediatric ward. In addition, communication skills can be improved. There are several methods:

  ◆ The easiest to master is the art of listening, then briefly repeating in your own words what was said. Especially in

PRACTICAL POINTS TO PONDER

Manage Your Stress

  ◆ *If you will learn to manage stress better, you will be able to take control of your life.*
  ◆ *Exercise is the best short-term stress reducer.*
  ◆ *Spend five minutes writing down the things that are most important in your life. Compare that with the things you spend most of your time doing. Cut back if you are doing things that aren't important.*
  ◆ *Join a group, any group!*
  ◆ *Use the power of love, whether in a religious, platonic, or romantic sense, to get you through the hard times.*
  ◆ *Practice stress management for one hour daily to reverse your heart disease!*

emotionally charged situations, such as with family, this method can be helpful. It tends to slow down and focus verbal communication, and enhances "body language" or nonverbal communication.

♦ Another communication skill to master is that of speaking about feelings rather than thoughts. We spend a lifetime learning to "edit" before we speak, making assumptions (or guesses) which may be incorrect. These usually are spoken as "thoughts." "I think you are angry" and "I think you need to rest" are examples of speaking thoughts. In times of stress, try speaking feelings, such as "I am angry, happy, embarrassed, lonely, worried, insecure, or sad." Then ask your loved one to respond similarly. (No fair trying "I feel you need a psychiatrist"!). This method can help get to the root of the situation or problem, thus opening up discussion. At the very least, it will clean up the line of communication, so that both parties are on the same wavelength. It takes openness and practice to speak feelings, and this, too, indicates willingness to have a dialog rather than the usual shouting match.

For some other ideas on stress, refer to "Thirty-five Ways to Leave your Stress" in chapter 8.

ANXIETY is commonly reported to cause distress and lack of satisfaction. In contemporary society there is much to make us anxious. Anxiety can escalate to the point of discomfort, causing withdrawal from many social situations, which is not good for mental health. It can also be frightening, as the symptoms of an anxiety or panic attack can mimic heart attack, with chest pressure, shortness of breath, rapid heart beat, and sweating.

Besides meditation, there are several helpful techniques which alleviate anxiety. The quieting response (see chapter 8) is effective to physically use reflexes to relax both the body and the mind. The body stress scanning technique (also chapter 8) is also effective. We urge you to learn and practice both these techniques often.

There is a group of behaviors, termed "learned behavior" (or Type A behavior), that seem to trap people on the treadmill of work. Often initiated at an early age (some experts say inborn), the typical pattern is a relentless, unyielding work ethic. Pretty good for business? However, after the first years of accomplishment, praise, promotion, and reward, these people don't seem to be able to "slow down and smell the roses." Often there is tension between spouses, but the Type A may not understand why (even after the umpteenth missed dinner). Life to them is competition, and slowing down or vacationing means falling behind. They thrive on pressure, deadlines, and challenges. Some, when the inevitable heart attack comes, don't want to be hospitalized, or after the first day begin to doubt they need care ("I must have had bad heartburn!"). Occasionally, the Type A will insist on doing push-ups at the bedside, while hooked up to the monitor, to prove everything is OK!

There is more to life than work, even for the long-term Type A personality. Often the best therapy is a close examination of goals. However, before this can be accomplished, the merry-go-round must stop. But how?

Strange as it may seem, there are few of us who have control of our own minds. With practice, the worries, schedules, and demands that keep the mind working overtime can be pushed out. Control of the mind during meditation allows for relaxation of the body, also. Relaxation and control. Together, they bring peace of mind (or inner peace). Many find it easier to discern the true goals in their lives after meditation.

ANGER is often found in people with heart or other serious disease. It is as if, instead of screaming, these people keep anger inside, till they (and their arteries) burst. Anger can and does come out eventually, but often is aimed at the ones closest to us. Anger is a strong emotion. Anger can also mask depression.

Talking about anger, directing it appropriately, and understanding where it came from sometimes help it be released, from inside. This can be a very gratifying experience. More about anger and how to deal with it is available in chapter 8.

FATIGUE is a symptom of many things: burn-out, insomnia, inability to cope, and depression. Sometimes it simply comes from prolonged inactivity.

DEPRESSION is very detrimental to performance, in business and at home. This unfortunate disease can be a block to reaching your goals: happiness, health, vigor, love. Depression drags down the mind and body. It actually inhibits the normal functioning of body tissues. Other symptoms of depression are change in appetite, insomnia, inability to feel pleasure, helplessness, and hopelessness. Depression is a common ailment, affecting up to 20 percent of Americans. If this sounds like you, let your personal physician know. There are many treatments which can help you remove this blockage, and help you heal the blockage in your heart. Read about them in chapter 8. The treatment is available, and it works. There is no reason to continue to feel this way!

It is a fact of our modern American society that many women and men have been victimized sexually, physically, and emotionally. This can leave deep scars and memories, some of which may not be conscious. This can adversely affect us in our later years as the scars open up. Heart disease may bring them out into the open. Maladaptive behavior, learned to cope with prior abuse, is often used to endure. By recognizing that the abuse was actual and real, and then (thankfully) leaving it in the past, present day happiness and peace can be a realistic goal.

The stress reduction component of our program would not be complete without group support. We spend several hours a week in our group at the Preventive Health Institute. It can be a valuable learning and healing tool. Group support can be as straightforward as an invitation to a fat-free meal! Often, groups evolve into "networks" for exercise and social life. Some even take the step of giving counsel and love to members in distress. Don't forget that word, love. It can be a lifesaver. Freud said, "the purpose of life is to love and to work." Many great philosophers and religious leaders have recognized the power of love to overcome obstacles. Don't downplay love's ability to get you through.

You are urged to join group sessions in your community. None available locally? Write the Preventive Health Institute for information on how to start a group. (Preventive Health Institute, 2130 Hollowbrook, Colorado Springs, CO 80918; 719/590-7037) Others have found this the single most helpful intervention they can make in their lifestyle.

Exercise—Move Your Body

Most of aging is really disuse. As the saying goes, "if you don't use it, you lose it." This is true, but you can gain some of it back. This takes exercise, however, about 30 minutes most every day.

Learn how to exercise the easy way in chapter 9.

Exercise can help your heart in several ways. The muscles of the extremities, with daily use, develop greater capacity to pull oxygen from the blood. The mitochondria (power plants) of the muscle hypertrophy, and the muscle becomes more efficient. (At this stage of life, don't expect to see too much enlargement of your muscles.) This causes beneficial effects in energy and vigor, even without any changes in the heart.

In addition, exercise will affect the heart and lungs. Weight loss makes it easier to move. Just as for other muscles, the heart and diaphragm muscles will respond by becoming more efficient. The heart benefits directly by having more oxygen supply. Although you should notice beneficial effects within two weeks, it is extremely important to start low and go slow. Don't overdo the first day. When you wake up the next day, soreness may cause you to call off the whole program. Remember, you are in this for the long haul. This is called pleasurable risk reduction.

STRETCHING can help prevent soreness. It is also important as a warm-up. This slowly stimulates the heart, allowing compensation to occur. (For those of you with angina pectoris, you know the initial morning walk can bring it on. Then, after rest and compensation occur, exercise can continue for much longer without symptoms.) The best resource is the book *Stretching* by Bob Anderson. Try several stretches, very slowly.

When your muscles are warmed up, it is time to start the aerobic part of exercise. (See chapter 9 for the exact "exercise prescription.") Eventually try to work up to 30 minutes most every day, but initially, remember to start low and go slow. Follow the parameters of the exercise prescription. Many people settle on walking as the optimal exercise because of convenience, but feel free to experiment with other equipment or sports. Water sports are a good alternative, especially if arthritis, weight, or weather are factors.

PRACTICAL POINTS TO PONDER

Exercise!

- *"No pain, no gain" is a myth. If you hurt, see your doctor. Something may be wrong.*
- *The most danger from an exercise program is at the very beginning. Be careful! Start out low and slow and gradually build up.*
- *Aerobic exercise should be a priority to prevent and reverse heart disease. Strength training is fine if you have more time.*
- *Most people settle on walking for 30 minutes most every day. Variety is the spice of life, so have a backup if you feel stale or the weather turns ugly. Try swimming, rowing, or biking for variety!*
- *Move your body for 30 minutes daily to reverse your heart disease.*

The last part of the exercise program is the cool-down. As the body exercises, blood vessels dilate and "energizing" (fight or flight) hormones are released. The cool-down allows these changes to reverse slowly. Some exercisers get dizzy if they skip the cool-down. The main reason for the cool-down, though, is to avoid changes in the rhythm of the heart (arrhythmias) from the high levels of hormones.

Many people are afraid that exercise, especially after a heart attack, will hurt them. While it is prudent to start low and slow, your heart, body, and mind desperately need exercise. Far from causing harm, exercise strengthens the heart and helps longevity. Use it or lose it!

If you have adverse effects from exercise, modifications can be made immediately. "Warnings" (chapter 9) can be used as a guide. Most people will notice one to two weeks of pleasant relaxation when they start an exercise program. This soon changes into a phase of increased energy and vigor, which will stay with you as long as you continue the program. The rise in endorphins causes these positive mental and physical benefits.

Most complaints about exercise are about time. Pick a time of day and stick to it. Form a habit. Practice, practice, practice, and soon you will enjoy. Exercise will be a routine part of your day, like eating and sleeping.

Look for further suggestions in chapter 9 for the practical way to start an exercise program.

CHAPTER FOUR

EATING RIGHT, THE PRACTICAL GUIDE

"You are what you eat."

We pride ourselves on giving practical advice. So let's analyze where you are, and explain where you should be. Then we can help you along the way!

What You Will Find in this Chapter

- Ten Steps to Heart Healthy Eating (page 52)
- Rate Your Diet (page 53)
- SAD (Standard American Diet) (page 57)
- What Is a 10 Percent Fat Meal Plan? (page 60)
- Changing Your Way of Thinking (page 61)
- Planning Ahead for a Fat-Free Kitchen (page 63)
- Cutting the Salt (page 67)
- Keeping Vitamins in Your Food (page 68)
- Recipe Substitutions (page 69)
- In Place of Meat: Where's the Beef? (page 71)
- Beans About Beans (page 72)
- Shortcuts to Vegetarian Eating (page 74)
- Controlling the Hunger Monster (page 75)
- Recipe Make-Overs (page 77)

Ten Steps to Heart Healthy Eating

1. HAVE A CLEAR IDEA OF YOUR OVERALL GOAL. Substitute some other food for one cheeseburger a week? Expect very slight improvement. Big change, big improvement!

2. HAVE A CLEAR IDEA OF WHICH FOODS CONTAIN FAT. Read the section on food labels, in chapter 5. The Department of Agriculture does not require meat, chicken, or milk products to have labels, yet they are all very high in fat!

3. TEST YOURSELF ON YOUR KNOWLEDGE OF NUTRITION. (Take the Rate Your Diet survey, which starts on the next page.)
    Aim for a total of about 20 grams of fat a day, which is about 10 percent of calories from fat.

4. CLEAN OUT THE KITCHEN OF FOODS YOU DO NOT WANT TO EAT. Removing temptation is easier than fighting temptation!

5. TAKE THE SHOPPING LIST ("HEALTHY FOODS SHOPPING LIST FOR EATING RIGHT," CHAPTER 5) AND LOAD UP ON STAPLES. You may want to get some nonstick cookware.

6. REVIEW CHAPTER 14, MENUS AND RECIPES. Pick out 10 and try them! Keep experimenting. Stay receptive to new foods and combinations.

7. PLAN AHEAD! Read about how to control the Hunger Monster (page 75) and dining out fat-free (chapter 6). Think about ways to handle situations you will find yourself in at a party or a restaurant.

8. REVIEW WHAT A SAD DIET MOST AMERICANS EAT (SAD, PAGE 57).

9. GET TO KNOW "BEANS ABOUT BEANS," PAGE 72. Beans are filling, inexpensive, tasty, and a great source of protein and fiber. Then find out what to do about gas.

10. EAT TO YOUR HEART'S CONTENT. You will improve your heart health, cure heartburn, and never worry about hunger. Enjoy!

Rate Your Diet

What type of ground beef did you eat last week?

Regular hamburger (30% fat)	0 points	_____
Lean ground beef, lamb (25% fat)	1 point	_____
Extra lean pork, veal (20% fat)	2 points	_____
Ground sirloin or round (10% fat)	3 points	_____
Healthy Choice ground beef	4 points	_____
I rarely eat meat, pork, or veal	5 points	_____

What did you eat for breakfast yesterday?

Bacon, eggs, sausage, fried potatoes, biscuits and gravy, sausage biscuit	0 points	_____
Often skip breakfast	1 point	_____
Egg McMuffin	3 points	_____
Pancakes and syrup	4 points	_____
Cereal, skim milk, orange juice, fruit, bagel	5 points	_____

What did you eat for lunch yesterday?

Big Mac, Whopper, fried fish/chicken	0 points	_____
Often skip lunch	1 point	_____
Lunch meat sandwich	2 points	_____
Low-fat tuna sandwich, 95% lean meat	3 points	_____
Peanut butter sandwich or bean burrito, chicken breast or fish (not fried)	4 points	_____
Baked potato with broccoli or bean soup	5 points	_____

What did you eat with lunch?

      French fries, onion rings, chips   0 points _____

      Low-fat chips, low-fat cookies or crackers   3 points _____

      Pretzels, rice cakes, fat-free chips   4 points _____

      Fruit or vegetables, salad, vegetable soup   5 points _____

What type of main dish did you eat for dinner yesterday?

      Ribs, steak, pork chops or similar, pizza   0 points _____

      Hot dogs, hamburgers, fried food   2 points _____

      Ate dinner out—not low fat   2 points _____

      Fish, chicken breast, other lean meat   4 points _____

      Pasta with marinara sauce, beans, tofu   5 points _____

How often do you eat out?

      Once or more daily   0 points _____

      Three to four times per week   1 point _____

      Once or twice a week   2 points _____

      Once or twice a month   4 points _____

      Rarely   5 points _____

Which meat/protein did you eat yesterday? (Multiply number of servings by number of points.)

      Cheese, eggs, liver, heart, brains   0 points _____

      High fat cuts of beef, lamb, pork or ham 0 points _____

      Beef round, pork loin, lean ham   1 point _____

      Veal, venison, elk, fish, chicken breast   3 points _____

      Beans, legumes, tofu, egg white,

          fat-free cheese, other vegetarian entrée 5 points _____

What kind of milk do you use?

      Whole milk (4% fat)   0 points _____

      Low-fat milk (2% fat)   1 point _____

      1% milk   3 points _____

      1% soy milk   4 points _____

      Skim milk (0% fat)   5 points _____

Which desserts did you eat yesterday?
Premium ice cream   0 points _____
Chocolate, cake, cookies, pie,
    regular ice cream, tofutti   1 point _____
Ice milk, frozen yogurt, sherbet,
    low-fat cookies   3 points _____
Fat-free desserts   4 points _____
Fruit   5 points _____

What types of cheese did you eat last week?
Cheddar, Swiss, Jack, Brie,
    American, cream cheese   0 points _____
Part skim mozzarella, Lappi, light cream
    cheese, light cheese, feta, farmer's   2 points _____
Any cottage cheese   4 points _____
Any fat-free cheese   5 points _____

How many eggs did you eat last week?
Six or more whole eggs   0 points _____
Three to six whole eggs   1 point _____
Egg Beaters, Scramblers, Second Nature,
    Egg Lights   4 points _____
Egg whites only—unlimited number   5 points _____

Which toppings did you use yesterday?
Sour cream, whipping cream, half & half   0 points _____
Light sour cream, Cool Whip Lite   3 points _____
Nonfat yogurt, nonfat sour cream   5 points _____

What kind of fat did you cook with yesterday?
Butter, Crisco, lard, bacon grease, chicken fat 0 points _____
Stick margarine   1 point _____
Tub margarine, olive oil, canola oil   3 points _____
Light margarine   4 points _____
None, cooking spray, fat-free spread   5 points _____

How much added fat did you eat yesterday (i.e. peanut butter, nuts, margarine, mayo, salad dressing)?

8-10 tsp. or more (average on salad)	0 points	_____
6-7 tsp. (average oil for cooking)	1 point	_____
2-3 tsp. (margarine on toast or potato)	2 points	_____
1-2 tsp. (average cream in coffee)	3 points	_____
I don't add fat	5 points	_____

What kind of salad dressing did you use last week?

Real mayo	0 points	_____
Miracle Whip, blue cheese, Russian	1 point	_____
Ranch, French, Thousand Island, creamy Italian, lite mayonnaise	2 points	_____
Vinegar and oil, Italian	3 points	_____
Miracle Whip Light, any light dressing	4 points	_____
Fat-free, vinegar, lemon juice, none	5 points	_____

What type of baked goods did you eat yesterday?

Pie, cake with icing, donut, muffin	0 points	_____
Coffee cake, sweet roll, french toast	1 point	_____
Granola bar, flour tortilla	3 points	_____
Bread, bagels, corn tortilla	4 points	_____
Oil free bread, low-fat bagel, pita bread	5 points	_____

What did you eat for snacks yesterday?

Chocolate, nuts, fatty dessert	0 points	_____
Potato chips, nuts, corn chips	1 point	_____
Buttery crackers, popcorn with fat	2 points	_____
Light popcorn, low-fat crackers or cookies	4 points	_____
Pretzels; angel food cake; fat-free cookies, crackers, or chips; sorbet	5 points	_____

How many pieces of fruit or cups of real fruit juice did you eat
yesterday? Add 1 point per piece: _____

How many servings of vegetables did you eat yesterday? Add 1
point per piece: _____

How many cups of legumes (fat-free refried beans, split peas,
navy beans, lentils, meatless chili, etc.) did you eat yesterday?
Add 2 points per serving: _____

How many servings of each did you have of these yesterday?
Wheat germ, brown rice, bulgur, cracked wheat, barley, quinoa,
corn, white or sweet potato, whole grain cereal or bread, corn
tortillas. Add 2 points per serving: _____

How many servings of crackers, popcorn, bagels, pretzels, white
bread, flour tortillas, white rice, or pasta did you eat yesterday?
Add 1 point per serving: _____

SCORE:
   100 points or more ...... Excellent low-fat eating.
   75 to 100 points .... On the right track.
   50 to 75 points .... Read this chapter carefully.
   Fewer than 50 points .. Better get serious about your heart!

SAD (Standard American Diet)

The Standard American Diet is promoted on TV and radio, in
magazines, and in restaurants. (Reference 26) It averages:
   ◆ Fat = 40 to 45%
   ◆ Carbohydrate = 20 to 30%
   ◆ Protein = 25 to 40%

Do you recognize the SAD advertisements? The industry spends $60 billion a year to entice you!

- "Beef, it's what's for dinner" by the American Beef Council.
- "Milk, it makes a body strong" by the Dairymen's Association.
- "Pork, the other white meat" by the Pork Producers.

WHAT DOES THE STANDARD AMERICAN DIET GET US?

- The highest rates of heart disease in the world. In non-Westernized countries, heart disease is much less frequent. As countries take on Western characteristics, the rate of heart disease rises. For example, the Japanese culture was studied. In Japan, heart disease was lowest, but Japanese natives who had moved to Hawaii had intermediate rates. In San Francisco, the heart disease rate among Japanese equaled that of native Americans.
- Very high rates of certain cancers: colon, breast, prostate. Again, only the United States has these high rates. So-called "underdeveloped countries" have much lower rates of these cancers.
- Food allergies
- Additives
- Bacterial contamination of our foods, especially from the sea. Each year, the number of deaths and illnesses from contamination rises.

American Heart Association Diet

The AHA diet is the standard "therapeutic" diet used by American doctors and dietitians. It recommends an eating plan consisting of:

- Fat = 30%
- Carbohydrate = 50 to 60%
- Protein = 10 to 20%

It is usually prescribed in less than one hour with a Registered Dietitian or about 10 minutes with a doctor! It takes an average of 10 hours to adequately learn a low-fat meal plan. It has become the "gold standard" for diet therapy, prior to drug prescription.

WHAT DOES THE AHA DIET GET US? Even though it is the gold standard, every control group in studies has steadily declined in health, and had increasing rates of atherosclerosis. The AHA diet is no better than SAD in preventing or reversing heart disease, diabetes, or obesity.

Healthy Heart Formula Meal Plan

Numerous studies have proven the ability of diet to prevent and reverse heart disease. It comes down to this:
- Fat = 10%
- Carbohydrate = 70 to 80%
- Protein = 10 to 20%

The Healthy Heart Formula meal plan contains most all the vitamins, minerals, trace elements, and antioxidants we need (except for vitamin E).

WHAT DOES THE HEALTHY HEART FORMULA MEAL PLAN GET US?
- Reversal of pre-existing heart disease
- Improvement and reversal of diabetes
- Weight loss may be a side effect
- Improvement of hypertension, the silent killer
- Lowering of cholesterol, even in those with genetically high cholesterol
- Cancer prevention
- Prevention of constipation, diverticulosis, hemorrhoids, and many other rectal problems
- Increased energy and vigor
- Less food allergy, less spastic colon

◆ No hunger, no yo-yo dieting. Most can eat as much as they are used to!

It really is SAD that you are hurting yourself with food. Break out of the cage of advertising in which you live. The world is a grand buffet of delicious and exciting foods. Try this plan to eat, drink, and be merry!

What Is a 10 Percent Fat Meal Plan?

The following tables were calculated for average people with average activity levels.

10% FAT MEAL PLAN FOR MEN

WEIGHT IN LBS	CALORIES	GRAMS OF FAT
100	1200	13
125	1500	16
150	1800	20
175	2100	23
200	2400	26
225	2700	30
250	3000	33

10% FAT MEAL PLAN FOR WOMEN

WEIGHT IN LBS	CALORIES	GRAMS OF FAT
90	990	11
100	1100	12
125	1375	15
150	1650	18
175	1925	21
200	2200	24
225	2475	27
250	2750	30

If you want to reverse heart disease, keep your fat intake at 61 the recommended 10 percent or less of total calories. This is how we derived the 10 percent fat meal plans:

- ◆ **For men:** weight in pounds x 12 = calories a day
- ◆ **For women:** weight in pounds x 11 = calories a day
- ◆ Calories a day x 10% = calories from fat
- ◆ Calories from fat divided by 9 = grams of fat
- ◆ **Note:** If you are not overweight or are extremely active, you may need more calories.

Changing Your Way of Thinking

WHERE TO BEGIN? Most of us are very set in our ways when it comes to food. You may have had some experiences that reinforced a typical high-fat diet. Just offer someone fat-free food and they may decline (even if the food is delicious). Have you

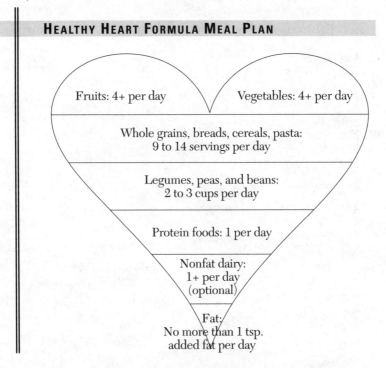

HEALTHY HEART FORMULA MEAL PLAN

Fruits: 4+ per day

Vegetables: 4+ per day

Whole grains, breads, cereals, pasta: 9 to 14 servings per day

Legumes, peas, and beans: 2 to 3 cups per day

Protein foods: 1 per day

Nonfat dairy: 1+ per day (optional)

Fat: No more than 1 tsp. added fat per day

FOOD FOR THOUGHT

- ◆ *Do you think what you eat can have an effect on your health?*
- ◆ *What would encourage you to change what you eat?*
- ◆ *Do you read food labels?*
- ◆ *What do carbohydrates do in the body? (See page 39 for more information.)*
- ◆ *What is the function of protein (amino acids) in the body? (See page 38 for more information.)*
- ◆ *What is the function of fat (oil) in the diet?(See page 35 for more information.)*
- ◆ *What is fiber (roughage)? (See page 40 and page 203 for more information.)*
- ◆ *Do you know any restaurants locally that offer heart healthy meals? When you dine out, is it an opportunity to splurge?*
- ◆ *Do you frequently dine at "all you can eat" restaurants? (See chapter 6 for information on dining out fat-free.)*
- ◆ *If you are "being good" about a diet, do you frequently feel hungry?*
- ◆ *What changes do you want from your food choices in the next year?*

Please review this quiz with your doctor or dietitian, then set a goal:

THE FIRST CHANGE IN MY DIET I WILL MAKE IS:

_____

_____

_____

_____

_____

_____

_____

Good luck! Now, take what you've learned from this quiz to care for your heart.

bought something labeled fat free at the grocery store and been 63
sorely disappointed? Unfortunately, it only takes one bad experience to "turn off" to a whole category of foods.

The good news is there are many great tasting fat-free and
low-fat foods available. See the recommendations in "The Best
Fat-Free and Low-Fat Foods," chapter 6.

Cooking fat free is the same. If you have tried one or two
recipes that didn't quite meet your standards, you may have said,
"This fat-free cooking is for the birds," and gone on with your
regular way of cooking. However, there are many tricks to fat-
free cooking and we've provided them in a step-by-step way to
make it easy to get started.

We only ask one thing—make the change! Change your way
of thinking about food. Leave all those preconceived ideas about
vegetarian, fat-free foods behind and open your mind to a way of
eating that is delicious, filling, and healthy! (It also just happens
to be low fat!) Try to broaden your repertoire of cooking to
include other ethnic foods such as Indian, Asian, and Middle
Eastern. Since these cultures are mostly vegetarian, some of the
most wonderful meatless dishes come from these countries.

Eat to live, rather than live to eat.

Planning Ahead for a Fat-Free Kitchen

GETTING STARTED You've decided to make the change—where do
you begin when it comes to food? Just taking the meat off your
plate won't be enough. You have to add more of the "good
stuff"—pasta, potatoes, vegetables, whole grains, fruit, legumes.
Here is a step-by-step plan for arranging your kitchen and your
life around your new fat-free but taste-full lifestyle!

Take an inventory of your kitchen. Get rid of all the high-fat
foods you will be tempted to eat. For a list of the foods you'll
want to keep on hand, see the shopping list in chapter 5.

COOKING EQUIPMENT/METHODS Please take a look at *how* you cook. (If the word "cook" is also a foreign term, turn to convenience foods and dining out in chapter 5 and chapter 6.) Does sautéing or frying come to mind? These are quick cooking methods, no doubt, but let's try to broaden our cooking methods to include fast, convenient, and more healthful ways of cooking. Here's a list of equipment for cooking quick, fat-free meals:

- ◆ Steamer for the stove or microwave
- ◆ Pressure Cooker
- ◆ Crockpot
- ◆ Stir Fry Wok
- ◆ Food Processor/Vegetable Chopper-Slicer
- ◆ Nonstick Sauté Pans
- ◆ Blender/Food Processor
- ◆ Deep Freezer
- ◆ Breadmaker. Imagine waking up to the smell of homemade cinnamon or hearty sourdough bread every morning! This is possible with a countertop breadmaker. Fresh bread doesn't need to be slathered in margarine to taste great—it's wonderful all by itself. Remember that bread isn't something to skimp on, it's something to base your diet on!

Condiments—Spice It Up!

If the spices you use are limited to salt, pepper, garlic salt, and cinnamon, then you need to spice up your cooking! When you take out the fat, you will need to add more spices for flavor. Spices add no fat, cholesterol, calories, or sodium—what a bargain! Keep in mind that spices lose their taste rather quickly so it's best to keep them for just six months. Some natural food stores sell spices in bulk so you can buy just the amount you need.

If buying fresh herbs, wrap them in a damp paper towel and place in a zip-lock plastic bag in your refrigerator to keep fresh. Or start your own windowsill herb garden for really fresh herbs!

Herbs and Suggested Uses

ALLSPICE: Traditionally used in spice cakes, pumpkin pies, etc., it is a blend of cloves, cinnamon, and nutmeg. Try it in sweet potatoes, stews, and soups.

BASIL: Though Italian cooking comes to mind, basil is actually used in Mexican, Indian, Greek, and Middle Eastern cuisines. Fresh basil goes well in salads and sauces and on pizza.

CARAWAY SEED: Those little seeds found in rye breads also go well in cabbage and noodle dishes.

CAYENNE PEPPER: In general, just a pinch is wise!

CINNAMON: The spice everyone has—but have you ever thought about using it in green beans or squash or a spicy bean soup?

CILANTRO: It is great in fresh salsas, salads, and sauces.

CELERY SEED: Traditionally used in coleslaw, but also good in soups and stews.

CORIANDER: The seeds are available whole or in powder form. Try it in curries, sweet dishes, and pasta salad.

CUMIN: Try it in chilis, soups, beans, and sauces.

CURRY: A blend of several herbs. Use it in creamy sauces, traditional curries, in beans, and in soups.

CARDAMOM: Try Basmati rice with cardamom seeds. The Basmati rice has a distinctive nutty flavor and the cardamom seeds give it a wonderful fragrance and taste. Also try in punches and cakes.

DILL WEED: It is great in sauces for vegetables. It's also good with grains and in salad dressing and dip mixes. This is an easy spice to grow.

FENNEL SEED: If you like Italian sausage, fennel is one of the predominant spices. Put it in lasagna, vegetarian burgers, and bean loafs to get the same flavor.

GARLIC: When in doubt, add garlic! Garlic powder can be used instead of fresh garlic—1/4 teaspoon for each garlic clove. Another shortcut is to buy chopped garlic in a jar. Garlic has been shown to lower cholesterol if you eat it daily.

GINGER: Gingerroot is common in Asian and Indian cooking. It can be used in marinating, in stir-fries, and in sauces. A shortcut to using it fresh is using a garlic press or grating it. Keep what you don't use in the freezer. Or buy it in a jar. Dried ginger is used in gingerbread and in sweet vegetables like squash, sweet potatoes, and carrots.

MINT: Sure, this is good in iced tea, but it also works well in Indian, Thai, and Vietnamese dishes. It often is used as a contrast to hot spices.

NUTMEG: Gives a nice touch to cream sauces and vegetables. Nutmeg is best bought as seeds and ground when you need it— similar to using a peppermill.

THE ONION FAMILY: Onions of all colors, garlic, chives, shallots, and scallions are members. Onion has been shown to lower cholesterol. When you take the fat out, you should add more onion for flavor. Experiment with different types!

SAFFRON: It gives taste to the Spanish dish, paella. Try it in rice, soups, and sauces.

The Mediterranean Family of Spices: Sage, Oregano, Rosemary, Thyme, Savory. These spices are often found together in Italian seasoning or in the French staple, Herbes de Provence. They are used alone or together in tomato sauces, vegetables, soups, stews, and stuffings.

Tarragon: Wonderful in cream sauces, salad dressings, and marinades.

Turmeric: Another herb that gives a yellow color and a pungent flavor to rice, vegetables, and Indian cuisine. It is used in curry.

Cutting the Salt

Switching to a plant-based diet automatically cuts a large amount of sodium you would be receiving in processed meats.

Many processed foods contain a significant amount of salt. Make sure to read the label to compare sodium content. Buy no-salt-added varieties of these foods when possible.

 ◆ Canned soups, vegetables, tomatoes, and tomato sauce
 ◆ Sauce mixes
 ◆ Teriyaki, soy, and stir-fry sauces
 ◆ Frozen dinners and vegetable dishes

Instead of using salt, there are many substitutes:

 ◆ Salt-free seasonings like Mrs. Dash
 ◆ If you just need to "shake something" but don't like the taste of salt substitutes, try Papa Dash light light salt. (1/4 the sodium of table salt)
 ◆ Lemon juice—a wonderful flavor enhancer
 ◆ Balsamic vinegar
 ◆ Malt vinegar
 ◆ Salt substitutes
 ◆ Garlic powder or fresh garlic
 ◆ More onion or fresh herbs

USING FRESH INGREDIENTS Use the freshest ingredients to add flavor as well as nutrients to your food. You may want to ask when your grocery gets their shipments of produce or of specific items. Planning your meals ahead of time (highly recommended) will help. In the summer, take advantage of farmer's markets that are often held several times a week. They guarantee (for the most part) the freshness of the produce. (Even at farmer's markets, some foods are from out of state, so ask.)

Organically grown produce is also often fresher and healthier, because preservatives aren't used. Fresh herbs add more flavor, which is why fine restaurants cook with them. Yes, they are more expensive, but think of how much your grocery bill has gone down now that you aren't buying all those expensive meats! Splurge a little to treat your taste buds. If you really want fresh produce, grow your own! This will also get you outdoors in the summer and you can really enjoy the fruits of your own labor.

PRACTICAL POINTS TO PONDER

Keeping Vitamins in Your Food

- *Buy fruits and vegetables as you need them. The longer they stay in your refrigerator, the more nutrients are lost.*
- *Eating raw fruits and vegetables is best! When cooking, cook in minimal amounts of water or steam. Thaw vegetables (like frozen spinach) instead of cooking them when putting in lasagna or a dip. Frozen vegetables going into salads can also be thawed instead of cooked.*
- *Don't wash produce until ready to eat or cook.*
- *Keep fruits and vegetables in produce drawer or if cooked, in opaque, airtight container.*
- *When possible, buy foods grown locally or from farmer's markets. This helps ensure freshness.*

GUIDE TO RECIPE SUBSTITUTIONS

FOR BAKING:

INSTEAD OF	USE
Oil	Applesauce, mashed banana, baby food prunes, or other baby food fruit
	Mashed sweet vegetable like carrots, sweet potatoes, or baby food
	Liquid butter buds, fat-free margarine (may not work in all recipes)
	Honey
One whole egg	1 mashed banana
	2 egg whites or 1/4 cup commercial egg substitute
	2 Tbsp. cornstarch or arrowroot
	1/4 cup tofu (blend with wet ingredients before adding to dry)
Butter or margarine in frosting	Marshmallow creme, fat-free cream cheese
Nuts	Grape nuts
	Smaller amounts of nuts and chopped more finely. Instead of cooking in the food, sprinkle small amount on top of food.

FOR COOKING:

Oil or margarine for sautéing	Nonstick spray
	Fat-free broth
	Wine, water, fruit juice, balsamic vinegar
	Liquid butter buds
Cream	Evaporated skim milk, plain yogurt, fat-free sour cream
	Vegetable purées
Sour cream	Plain nonfat yogurt, fat-free sour cream, puréed tofu
	Puréed fat-free cottage cheese plus lemon juice
Cream cheese	Fat-free cream cheese, or puréed fat-free ricotta or cottage cheese
Olives	Capers, pimientos
Regular cheese	Fat-free cheese—works best when mixed in a food like a casserole, or melted in, rather than melted on top
	Just a sprinkle of regular cheese—the sharper the flavor, the less you need to add a little zing
Baking chocolate	3 Tbsp. cocoa powder per ounce

At the Table

ON YOUR BREAD:

- If you buy fresh bread from a bakery or make your own, the bread is delicious with nothing on it!

FAT-FREE REPLACEMENTS FOR MARGARINE OR BUTTER:

- Promise Ultra fat-free margarine
- Roasted garlic (the longer cooked, the milder it gets)
- Honey or jam/fruit spread
- Fat-free cream cheese (flavor it by whipping in jam, honey, spice mixes, or some fat-free salad dressing mix)
- Fat-free Boursin Cheese Spread (page 217)

FILLINGS FOR SANDWICHES:

- Bean spread or Guiltless Gourmet fat-free bean dips
- Eggless egg salad (mashed firm tofu with fat-free mayo, relish, etc.)
- Fat-free cheese
- Tossed salad with fat-free cheese and dressing in pita pocket
- Leftover bean loaf
- Vegetarian burger (bought frozen and cooked in toaster-oven or microwave)
- Meatless Sloppy Joes (page 263)
- Roasted eggplant, zucchini, or peppers

IN PLACE OF HIGH-FAT SANDWICH SPREADS:

- Fat-free mayonnaise
- Dijon, yellow, German, or gourmet flavored mustard
- Fat-free "Dijonaise" (just mix a bit of fat-free mayo or mock mayo with Dijon to taste)
- Salsa
- Nonfat yogurt
- Ketchup (sounds a bit funny, but it's really good!)
- Fat-free honey Dijon, Italian, or ranch dressing

OTHER CONDIMENTS TO HAVE AVAILABLE:

+ Low-sodium soy sauce or tamari
+ Worcestershire sauce
+ Salsa
+ Chutney
+ Tabasco or Pick-a-Peppa sauce
+ Seasoning mix like Mrs. Dash, seasoned salt
+ Butter buds or Molly McButter (good for veggies, potatoes)
+ Cajun spice mix

IN PLACE OF MEAT: WHERE'S THE BEEF? If you like the texture of food you can "sink your teeth into," here are a few substitutes:

FOR GROUND BEEF:

+ *Grains* Bulgur, couscous, rice, oatmeal, and millet can be used in soups and chilis and with other vegetables and beans to make "burgers," loafs, and other generally meat-containing dishes.
+ *Eggplant* The texture of eggplant also imitates meat. Put it in casseroles, dips, and lasagna. Roasted, it is wonderful on pizza, in a sandwich, or stuffed in pita bread!
+ *Mushrooms* Have you seen those "Texas sized" mushrooms at your grocery? Called Portobello, this variety is big enough for a sandwich. Cook in wine and garlic and have in your sandwich or pasta. Or steam briefly in the microwave and grill them. Mushrooms can also be used in casseroles, sauces, and soups and in veggie burgers as a meat substitute.
+ *Seitan (wheat gluten)* This food is often called "wheat meat." It can be bought frozen in many different ways—in slices, chicken style, like a roast. It is found already marinated or seasoned in the refrigerated section at large natural food stores. See Faux Fajitas, page 254.
+ *Tofu* is made from soybeans in a process comparable to

making cheese. The beauty of tofu (and also the reason for its negative reputation) is that it does not have much flavor of its own. It takes on whatever flavor you choose to give it. Therefore it can be used in sizzling Chinese soups, in Southwest chili, as a meat substitute in tacos, as a cheese substitute in lasagna, as a substitute for eggs in "egg salad" or egg foo young. To make tofu have a meatier texture, freeze, then thaw and squeeze out excess water. It can be marinated and grilled. Tofu can also be used to make puddings and pies, dips, and sauces. Mori-Nu makes a new low-fat tofu that is vacuum packaged. It doesn't need refrigeration so you can stock your pantry. Tofu comes in different textures for many types of dishes.

◆ *Textured Vegetable Protein (TVP)* This is found in dry granules at the health food store, often in bulk. It works well when substituted for ground beef in soups, chilis, casseroles, and meat loafs.

◆ *Tempeh* is an Indonesian fermented soy product with a texture similar to meat. It can be used in casseroles and other dishes, and also can be used to make "burgers." Tempeh can also be found already marinated in different

BEANS ABOUT BEANS				
TYPE	**CALORIES IN 1/3 CUP**	**PROTEIN (GM)**	**FAT (GM)**	**CARBOS (GM)**
Pinto	75	4.9	0.3	13.6
Kidney	73	4.8	0.3	13.2
Garbanzo	80	4.5	1.1	13.5
Lentils	71	5.2	0.5	12.8
Navy	79	5.2	0.4	14.0
Lima	84	5.0	0.4	15.6
Black	75	4.9	0.3	13.6
Split pea	77	5.3	0.2	13.9
Soybean	78	6.6	3.4	6.5

ways such as Thai, fajita, "burger" patties, etc., at larger
health food stores.

◆ *Beans* All beans and peas also make great meat substitutes.
The more you learn about beans, the more you'll like
them! Check out the many great varieties. A great source
of protein, they taste wonderful, too!

INTESTINAL GAS If you rapidly increase your intake of beans, you
may notice a temporary increase in gas. Beans are a great source
of fiber, which makes you regular. Intestinal bacteria works to
break down sugar in the bean; the result is gas.

PRACTICAL POINTS TO PONDER

The Power of Plants

Plant products offer many benefits over animal products—
for what they don't have (saturated fat and cholesterol) and
for what they do have (phytochemicals and fiber). For
example, foods made from soybeans have been shown to
enhance health in several ways:

◆ *Soy protein (TVP, soy milk, tofu, soybeans) have been*
shown to reduce serum cholesterol. (Reference 31)

◆ *Eating soy protein instead of animal protein seems to*
affect how much calcium is lost from bone; an important
consideration for those concerned with osteoporosis.
(Reference 32)

◆ *In one study, women with the highest soy food consump-*
tion had less then half the risk of breast cancer than those
who eat soy rarely. Women with the lowest cancer rate
eat 2 ounces daily.

◆ *Other research showed that eating soybeans or tofu cut*
the risk of rectal cancer by more than 80 percent. Just
two servings of soy a week seemed to be protective.

Note that some soy products contain more fat than some
other plant products.

74 Your body rapidly adapts. Soaking, then rinsing beans also helps. The high fiber in foods like beans cures hemorrhoids and cuts your incidence of colon cancer!

Beano is a product to cut down on gas. It works! It breaks down the nonabsorbable chains of sugar into smaller, absorbable sugars. Besides less gas, the body absorbs more sugar calories. Less fiber is left in the colon.

Shortcuts to Vegetarian Eating

In the past, "in a hurry" meant calling out for pizza, going through the drive-through window for a burger, or just grabbing a doughnut or chocolate bar. You need to learn some healthier shortcuts. Here are a few tips that can save you time and fat!

MAKE EXTRA! The following recipes, found in chapter 14, all freeze well:

◆ Spinach Stuffed Shells
◆ Vegetarian Chili
◆ Bean and Rice Burritos
◆ Millet Burgers
◆ Crustless Quiche
◆ Lentil Soup

Other foods that freeze well include: pancakes, soups, casseroles, lasagna, muffins, chili, pasta dishes, and bean loaves.

USE LEFTOVERS CREATIVELY! If you plan ahead a bit, you can use leftovers in ways no one will suspect. Here are a few examples from the recipes in chapter 14:

◆ On Monday... Vegetarian Chili (page 231)
◆ On Tuesday... Minute Minestrone Soup (page 229)
◆ On Wednesday... Soft tacos with Monday's chili or taco salad with baked tortilla chips
◆ On Thursday... Use the leftover vegetables from Tuesday's soup to go in a curried rice dish

Controlling the Hunger Monster

◆ *Eat three meals and two snacks a day. Don't skip break-fast. Instead of letting hunger build all day, snacking prevents overeating in the evening. When you are extremely hungry, anything tastes good and temptation to eat junk food is greatest.*

◆ *Drink lots of water. At no calories, it's a bargain. Drink a glass before eating.*

◆ *Fat free goes a long way. At only 4 calories per gram of carbohydrate or protein, you don't have to be afraid of fat-free products in small amounts.*

◆ *Exercise, at a moderate intensity, helps to suppress the appetite. Exercise daily. Consider taking a short walk when hunger strikes.*

◆ *Plan ahead. Have snacks with you. Fruit and cut up vegetables are nutritious, healthy, satisfying, and guilt-free. Keep them available all day.*

◆ *We are more efficient when we snack. Studies on office workers and college students have proven that a mid-afternoon snack prevents the "blahs" and improves productivity and efficiency.*

◆ *Hunger is a message. Listen to why you eat. If the muscles need energy, feed them. However, if you are eating because you are angry, lonely, or depressed; you may want to do something about the emotions. Just because we learned a behavior like overeating doesn't mean it helps us adapt better.*

◆ *You can't live your life hungry. Learn to feed the hunger, be it physical or emotional.*

◆ *Get your fill of the other pleasures in life: love, sex, a job well done, runner's high, and more.*

◆ *Treat yourself to bite-sized portions. Often a little goes a long way to satisfy hunger.*

◆ On Friday... Mock Egg Foo Young

◆ On Saturday... Oriental burgers with Sweet and Sour Sauce (using leftover Mock Egg Foo Young patties)

◆ On Sunday... Pinto beans and texmati rice. On Sunday night... Seven layer bean dip with fat-free tortilla chips

BUY CANNED AND CONVENIENCE FOODS Keep on hand canned beans, fat-free broths, garlic in a jar, soup in a cup, tomatoes, vegetarian chilis, vegetarian burgers and hot dogs (remember that all vegetarian "look alikes" are not necessarily low fat!). In recipes, the canned foods will save you a lot of time. The convenience foods can be used to make instant meals. See "The Best Fat-Free and Low-Fat Foods" on page 95 and "Fifteen-Minute Meals" on page 209.

EASY SAUCES There are many sauces in jars and sauce mixes that are vegetarian and fat free. Chinese sweet and sour sauce, ginger and garlic sauce, "Chicken Tonight," and Hain fat-free brown gravy mix are just a few.

KEEP QUICK COOKING GRAINS ON HAND The old standby is brown rice which can take an hour to cook. Couscous takes 3 minutes. Bulgur and kasha can be cooked in 10 to 15 minutes or less. Many people prefer the taste of fresh pasta, which cooks in minutes. Grains can also be used as leftovers or cooked in bulk and frozen.

USE SPEEDY COOKING METHODS Bring out your pressure cooker and use it to cook beans and grains; it will cut your cooking time in half! Don't overlook the microwave for steaming vegetables and grains. A stir-fry meal is quick—especially if you use frozen prepared vegetables and fat-free prepared sauces.

Recipe Make-Overs

Learn how to take these typical recipes and turn them into a low-fat vegetarian feast! Here are a few examples:

LASAGNA original recipe *Serves:* 8

1 onion, chopped	1 garlic clove, chopped
1 Tbsp. oil	1 pound ground beef
1 package lasagna noodles	1 tsp. oil
1 tsp. salt	2 cups tomato sauce
1 pound mozzarella cheese,	1 pound cottage cheese
grated; 1/2 cup set aside	
4 oz. fresh grated Parmesan cheese	

Preparation:

1. Sauté onion and garlic in oil. Add ground beef. Cook until brown. Drain fat.
2. Cook noodles, adding oil and salt to water.
3. Layer noodles, sauce, ground beef, mozzarella, cottage cheese, and Parmesan, ending with sauce on top of the last layer of noodles. Sprinkle on reserved 1/2 cup mozzarella.

TO MODIFY THIS RECIPE:

There are several options for changing this recipe:

- Omit 1 pound ground beef and save 100 grams of fat!
- Use 1 cup of TVP hydrated in tomato juice or fat-free beef broth, 1 to 2 packages frozen spinach, cooked, with water squeezed out, or use sliced eggplant cooked and layered between noodles.
- Omit 1 Tbsp. oil and save 14 grams of fat!
- Cook the onion and garlic in broth, wine, or water instead.
- Instead of 1 pound regular mozzarella cheese, use fat-free cheese and save 60 grams of fat!
- Instead of 4 ounces fresh grated Parmesan cheese, use 1 Tbsp. and save 28 grams of fat!

◆ Instead of 1 pound regular cottage cheese, use fat-free ricotta or cottage cheese and save 20 grams of fat!

OTHER INGREDIENTS TO ADD...

◆ Add more onion and garlic than called for to spice it up. Add more veggies to the tomato sauce, such as chopped bell peppers, sun dried tomatoes, fresh herbs, and chopped zucchini. Even if you use bottled tomato sauce, you can still "doctor" it up.

TOTAL FAT SAVED: 222 GRAMS FOR ENTIRE RECIPE OR 28 GRAMS PER SERVING!

CHILI original recipe *Serves: 8*

1 large onion	1 large green pepper
2 Tbsp. oil	2 pounds lean ground beef
28 oz. can tomato sauce	16 oz. can tomato sauce
2 Tbsp. chili powder	1 teaspoon salt
15 oz. can kidney beans	8 oz. cheddar cheese, grated
Tortilla chips	

Preparation:

1. Using a large pot, sauté onion and pepper in oil until tender.
2. Add ground beef and cook, stirring often, until brown.
3. Add tomatoes, tomato sauce, seasoning, and beans. Simmer slowly for 45 minutes.
4. Serve topped with cheddar cheese and with tortilla chips.

TO MODIFY THIS RECIPE:

There are several options for changing this recipe:
◆ Omit ground beef and save 173 grams of fat!
◆ Use rehydrated TVP , or a mix of bulgur and beans and other grains. Some use soy grits or brown rice to add texture. You can also use crumbled firm tofu, chopped seitan, or tempeh.

◆ Omit oil and save 28 grams of fat!
◆ Sauté in broth, wine, or tomato juice.
◆ Omit regular cheddar cheese and save 72 grams of fat!
◆ Use fat-free cheddar or mozzarella instead.
◆ Omit regular tortilla chips and save 72 grams of fat!
◆ Use baked tortilla chips instead. Make your own or try Baked Tostitos.

INGREDIENTS TO INCREASE:

◆ Onion, green pepper, and seasonings. You may want to use different varieties and colors of beans.

TOTAL FAT SAVED: 345 GRAMS FOR ENTIRE RECIPE OR 43 GRAMS PER SERVING!

CHAPTER FIVE

THE FAT-FREE EATER'S GUIDE TO THE GROCERY STORE

"Education is not preparation for life; education is life itself."
—John Dewey

Ten Ways to Shop Smart

Lost? Think Olestra is good for you? Is vegetarian fat free? This chapter is for you. Learn which food will lower your cholesterol, just by eating it!

1. WRITE OUT A MENU OF PROPOSED MEALS FOR THE WEEK. Make a grocery list according to your menus.

2. IF YOU BUY FROM A FARMER'S MARKET OR FOOD CO-OP, SHOP THERE FIRST.

3. HAVE A SNACK BEFORE YOU GO. Better yet, go right after a meal. You'll spend more money (and buy things that may not be health-enhancing) if you are hungry.

4. MAKE SURE YOU HAVE TIME TO GO TO THE STORE. When you are in a hurry, you won't have time to check out the food labels.

5. TO ENSURE THAT YOUR DIET IS TOP-QUALITY, FILL MOST OF YOUR CART WITH THE BASICS—FRUITS, VEGETABLES, WHOLE GRAINS, BEANS. Convenience and processed foods should be a smaller percentage of what you buy.

6. LEAVE HOME ANYONE THAT MIGHT BE A HINDRANCE TO HEALTHY SHOPPING.
This includes children and spouses! On the other hand, it's never too soon (or too late) to teach the benefits of healthy eating. My 4 year old has already picked up the idea that too much fat isn't good for you. Since many of our "problem" eating habits are learned as children, I'm glad that he is learning healthy eating now.

7. EXPAND BEYOND THE FOODS YOU USUALLY BUY. Be adventurous. Go tropical!

8. READ THE LABEL TO AVOID FOODS THAT ARE HIGH IN FAT, SODIUM, AND OTHER INGREDIENTS YOU MAY BE TRYING TO AVOID.

9. ALWAYS BE ON THE LOOKOUT FOR NEW FAT-FREE PRODUCTS. If you hear of a new product but it isn't available at your store, ask the manager to order it for you.

10. DON'T OVERLOOK MAIL-ORDER FOR SOME VEGETARIAN AND FAT-FREE FOODS.
Vegetarian Times magazine regularly has listings of vegetarian products by mail.

Using the Food Label to Your Advantage

Just a few years ago, the food label was sabotaging the American public's good intentions to eat healthier. Confusing descriptions of food, claims that had no meaning, and serving sizes that were unrealistic made a trip to the grocery store more like a stint on a TV quiz show. (Find the truly low-fat food and you can take it home with you!)

However, all that changed when new food label laws were enacted. FDA Commissioner David Kessler describes the changes in food labeling: "The goal is simple: a label the public can understand and count on—that would bring them up to date with today's health concerns. It is a goal with three objectives:

First, to clear up confusion; second, to help us make healthy choices; and third, to encourage product innovation, so that companies are more interested in tinkering with the food in the package, not the words on the label."

Below is a sample of the new food label, which should be familiar to you by now.

THE NEW FOOD LABEL AT A GLANCE

Nutrition Facts

Serving Size 1 cup (248g)
Servings Per Container 4

Amount Per Serving

Calories 150   Calories from Fat 35

	% Daily Value*
Total Fat 4g	**6%**
Saturated Fat 2.5g	**12%**
Cholesterol 20mg	**7%**
Sodium 170mg	**7%**
Total Carbohydrate 17g	**6%**
Dietary Fiber 0g	**0%**
Sugars 17g	
Protein 13g	

Vitamin A 4%   •   Vitamin C 6%

Calcium 40%   •   Iron 0%

* Percent Daily Values are based on a 2,000 calorie diet. Your daily values may be higher or lower depending on your calorie needs:

	Calories:	2,000	2,500
Total Fat	Less than	65g	80g
Sat Fat	Less than	20g	25g
Cholesterol	Less than	300mg	300mg
Sodium	Less than	2,400mg	2,400mg
Total Carbohydrate		300g	375g
Dietary Fiber		25g	30g

Calories per gram:

Fat 9   •   Carbohydrate 4   •   Protein 4

Defining Descriptions Here are the definitions of claims you now see on the label.

Free: Contains either zero, a trivial amount, or an amount "physiologically inconsequential" of any of these components: fat, saturated fat, cholesterol, sodium, sugars, and calories. "Calorie free" means less than 5 calories per serving. "Sugar free" and "fat free" mean less than 0.5 gram per serving.

Low: This term can be used on foods that could be eaten frequently without exceeding dietary guidelines for one or more of: fat, saturated fat, cholesterol, sodium, and calories. Here are some examples:
- ◆ Low fat: 3 grams or less per serving
- ◆ Low saturated fat: 1 gram or less per serving
- ◆ Low sodium: less than 140 milligrams per serving
- ◆ Very low sodium: less than 35 milligrams per serving
- ◆ Low cholesterol: less than 20 milligrams per serving
- ◆ Low calorie: 40 calories or less per serving

High: One serving provides 20 percent or more of the Daily Value of a nutrient.

Good Source: One serving provides 10 to 19 percent of the Daily Value of a nutrient.

Reduced: The product is nutritionally altered and contains 25 percent less of a nutrient or calories than the regular or reference product.

Less: This product contains 25 percent or less of a nutrient or of calories than the regular or reference product. "Fewer" can be used instead of "less."

Light: Can mean two things:
   1. A nutritionally altered product containing a third fewer
      calories or half the fat of the reference food. If the food
      derives 50 percent or more of its calories from fat, the
      reduction must be 50 percent of the fat.
   2. The sodium content of a low-calorie, low-fat food has
      been reduced by 50 percent. "Light in sodium" may be
      used on foods in which the sodium content has been
      reduced by 50 percent.

More: Contains a nutrient that is at least 10 percent of the Daily
Value more than the reference food.

Percent Fat Free: Must meet definitions for low fat or fat free. If
a food contains 5 grams of fat per 100 grams, it must be labeled
"95% fat-free."

Healthy: To be labeled healthy, a product has to be low in fat, low
in saturated fat, limited in cholesterol and sodium, and provide
at least 10 percent of the Daily Value for vitamin A, vitamin C,
iron, calcium, protein, or fiber. Meal-type products like frozen
dinners must provide at least 10 percent of the Daily Value for
two or three nutrients, depending on the type and size of the
meal. Sodium limits will be phased in.

KEY CHANGES IN FOOD LABELS
   ◆ Labels contain nutrient information related to today's
     health concerns: fat, saturated fat, cholesterol, dietary
     fiber.
   ◆ Nutrient information is also shown as a percentage of
     Daily Value, a reference to show how a food fits into the
     total diet. Based on 2000 calories per day.
   ◆ New clearly-defined meanings for the words "light, low
     calorie, and high fiber."

◆ Claims about a relationship between a nutrient and a specific disease will be allowed. See list on page 88.

◆ Standardized serving sizes which make comparisons between similar products easier.

◆ Fruit juices and fruit drinks will have the percentage of fruit juice listed.

PRACTICAL POINTS TO PONDER

Label Logic

An easy way to put food labels to work for you:

◆ *Check out the serving size. All the information on the label is based on that serving size. If the serving size is 1/2 cup, but you'd typically eat 1 cup, you need to multiply all the nutrient information by two.*

◆ *Look at the fat grams. Ignore all the percentages for fat, saturated fat, cholesterol, etc. Remember those percentages are based on a 30-percent fat, 2000-calorie diet or 65 grams total fat. Your fat budget is about 20 grams, so you should just compare the total fat grams to your goal for the day. Aim for 5 grams of fat per meal with the extra 5 grams of fat dispersed between snacks throughout the day. With that in mind, if a food is to be the main dish or entree, 3 to 4 grams of fat would be acceptable. However if the food is just an accompaniment or side dish, look for foods with 0 to 2 grams of fat.*

◆ *Look at the saturated fat grams. All fats are a mixture of polyunsaturated, monounsaturated, and saturated. See page 36 to find out the typical amount of saturated fats in different oils and fat. By choosing the food with the lowest amount of fat, you will probably be getting the food with the least amount of saturated fat.*

◆ *Will extra fat be needed in the preparation of this food? Many times, the label lists fat for the packaged mix, but*

◆ "Standardized" products such as ice cream and
  mayonnaise were previously exempt from listing ingredients but will now be required to have an ingredient list.
◆ Voluntary nutrition information for many raw foods will be
  available at point of purchase site.
◆ Meat, dairy products, and seafood are still not required to
  have nutrition labeling.

Label Logic (continued)

*not as prepared. Also keep in mind that you should be
able to omit most oil or use the substitutions for fat listed
on page 69.*

◆ *Look at other nutrients on the label: sodium, fiber, and vitamins. Vitamins are given in percentages of Reference
  Daily Intakes or RDIs. Your fiber goal is 25 to 30 grams
  per day—an easy goal with the Healthy Heart Formula.
  Sodium intake should be below 2,400 milligrams per day.*

◆ *Remember that just because a product is vegetarian, it
  isn't necessarily low fat! Peanut butter is made from a
  plant but a majority of its calories come from fat!*

◆ *There may not be a nutrition label. You will find a large
  number of products made by small companies—they
  aren't required to have food labels. Look at the ingredient list, which lists ingredients in descending order by
  weight. Oil should be at the bottom of the list and defi-
  nitely not in the first half of ingredients. You can also
  check the ingredient list to find the type of fat used in the
  product.*

◆ *Remember that "fat free" doesn't mean "calorie free." Fat-
  free foods can be delicious—to the point that it may be
  hard to stop eating them! A friend of ours can eat a whole
  box of Snackwell's cookies! It could cause weight gain in
  sedentary folk!*

HEALTH CLAIMS ALLOWED ON THE PACKAGE

Saturated fat and cholesterol and coronary artery disease: Foods using this claim must also meet the definitions for "low fat," "low saturated fat" and "low cholesterol."

Fat and cancer: Foods using this claim must also meet the definition for "fat free."

Calcium and osteoporosis: Foods using this claim must have 20 percent or more of the Daily Value for calcium (200 milligrams per serving), have a calcium content that exceeds the food's content of phosphorous, and contain a form of calcium easily absorbed by the body. See calcium in foods on page 129.

PRACTICAL POINTS TO PONDER

Questions You May Have

◆ *When I looked at a label, the food was labeled "fat free" and there were 0 grams of fat but 4 calories from fat. How can the food be labeled fat free even though there are calories from fat?* The grams of fat listed are rounded off. Technically, if a product has 0.5 gram of fat or less, it can be called fat free. The grams of fat are rounded up or down, so to figure out exactly how much fat is in the product, divide the calories from fat by nine.

◆ *What should I think about a product that has 6 percent Daily Value for fat?* We suggest you ignore the percent Daily Value for fat, saturated fat, and cholesterol. Those numbers are based on a 2,000-calorie meal plan that contains 30 percent fat. The Healthy Heart Formula Meal Plan strives for 10 percent fat and may be higher or lower in calories. See page 60 for your suggested daily calories based on weight and sex.

Fiber-containing grain products, fruits, and vegetables, and cancer: Foods using this claim must meet the definition "fat free" and must naturally be a "good source" of fiber.

Fruits, vegetables, and grain products that contain fiber and risk of coronary heart disease: Must meet definition of "fat free," "low saturated fat," and "low cholesterol" and must naturally contain at least 0.6 grams soluble fiber per serving.

Sodium and hypertension (high blood pressure): Must meet definition of "low sodium."

Fruits and vegetables and cancer: Must meet definition for "fat free" and must naturally be a "good source" of either vitamin A, vitamin C, or dietary fiber.

Folic acid and neural tube defects: Food must be naturally high in folic acid, which has been proven to reduce spina bifida and other birth defects of the spinal canal.

EXCEPTIONS TO THE RULES:

As is true with most rules, there are exceptions:

- ◆ 2% milk can be called "low fat" even though it doesn't meet the low-fat definition of 3 grams of fat per serving. In fact, low-fat milk can contain up to 5 grams of fat per serving. Only buy skim milk!

These are exempt:

- ◆ Food produced by small companies.
- ◆ Foods served for immediate consumption—as on an airplane or in a restaurant.
- ◆ Ready-to-eat food that is not for immediate consumption—such as from a grocery deli or bakery.
- ◆ Plain coffee, tea, spices, and other foods that contain no significant amount of nutrients.

◆ The term "light" can still be used to describe texture and color as in "light brown sugar" or "light and fluffy."

◆ Food in small packages, like Life Savers, are not required to carry a food label. However, the phone number or address of the company must be listed so consumers can get nutrition information.

Healthy Foods Shopping List for Eating Right

This is a basic list to get you headed in the right direction. This may not be all you want to eat, but all these foods are good to your heart and help to prevent cancer. They are all very low in fat. You may notice unexpected weight loss if you stick to these foods only.

WHOLE GRAINS:

Amaranth	Barley	Buckwheat
Bulgur	Corn	Millet
Oats	Popcorn	Quinoa
Rice	Rye	Sorghum
Triticale	Wheat	Wheat berries

VEGETABLES:

Arugula (a green)	Asparagus	Bamboo shoots
Beets	Broccoli	Brussels sprouts
Burdock	Cabbage	Carrots
Cauliflower	Celery	Celery root
Chicory	Chile peppers	Cocozelle
Collard greens	Cucumbers	Daikon
Eggplant	Endive	Escarole
Jerusalem artichoke	Jicama	Kale
Leeks	Lettuce	Mushrooms
Mustard greens	Okra	Onions
Radishes	Rutabagas	Scallions
Spinach	Sprouts	Squash

Sweet potato
Turban squash
Watercress
Zucchini

Swiss chard
Turnips
White potato

Taro
Water chestnuts
Yams

FRUITS:

Apple
Blackberries
Carambola
Cherries
Dates
Grapes
Kiwifruit
Lichee
Loquat
Orange
Peach
Pineapple
Pomegranate
Quince
Strawberries
Tomato

Apricots
Blueberries
Casaba melon
Cranberries
Figs
Guava
Kumquat
Limes
Mango
Papaya
Pear
Plantain
Prune
Raisins
Tangelo
Watermelon

Banana
Cantaloupe
Cherimoya
Currants
Grapefruit
Honeydew melon
Lemon
Loganberries
Nectarine
Passion fruit
Persimmon
Plum
Pummelo
Raspberries
Tangerine

LEGUMES:

Azuki beans
Chick peas
Green peas
Lima beans
Pinto beans

Black beans
Fava beans
Kidney beans
Mung beans
Split peas

Black eyed peas
Garbanzo beans
Lentils
Navy Beans
White beans

PROTEIN FOODS:

Egg whites
Soy milk

Nonfat dairy products
Tempeh

Seitan
Tofu

BEVERAGES:

Fruit juice	Herbal teas	Vegetable juices
Seltzer	Skim milk	Water

DESSERTS AND SNACKS:

Ice cream substitutes: sorbet, fat-free yogurt, popsicles
Fat-free cakes and cookies: like Entenmann's, Snackwell's,
Health Garden, fat-free fig bars (Nabisco and Mother's)
See page 95 for "The Best Fat-Free and Low-Fat Foods."

Try different combinations and additions to give more variety.
Don't forget that the color, amount, presentation, and smell of
your food will enhance your enjoyment.

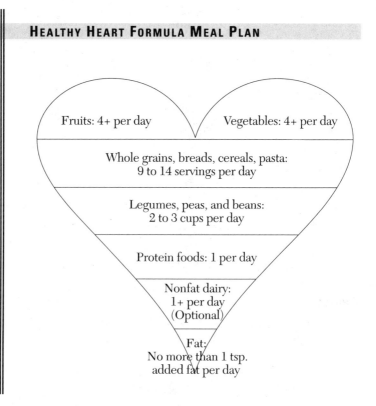

HEALTHY HEART FORMULA MEAL PLAN

Fruits: 4+ per day

Vegetables: 4+ per day

Whole grains, breads, cereals, pasta:
9 to 14 servings per day

Legumes, peas, and beans:
2 to 3 cups per day

Protein foods: 1 per day

Nonfat dairy:
1+ per day
(Optional)

Fat:
No more than 1 tsp.
added fat per day

Ingredient Guide to Vegetarian Eating

Miso, quinoa, seitan: A new language? No, just some of the new foods you might want to try on a health enhancing eating plan! Here is a guide to ingredients which may be new and different to you.

BUCKWHEAT/KASHA: Available as buckwheat flour, or groats; when groats are toasted it's called kasha. You may see kasha as a type of breakfast cereal in health food stores. Kasha has a hearty flavor and cooks rather quickly.

BULGUR: Use it in place of rice. It cooks quickly—with some types you just need to pour boiling water and let it sit.

CAPERS: Small buds that are usually pickled. They are great in salads and sauces and are a good substitute for olives on a vegetarian pizza.

CHICK PEAS: Also called garbanzo beans, you will frequently find them on salad bars. They make wonderful sandwich spreads, dips, and vegetarian burgers.

COUSCOUS: Traditionally made from crushed wheat, the couscous found in grocery stores is similar to a tiny pasta and is quick cooking.

LENTILS: A quick cooking legume that is very versatile. Red lentils cook even more quickly than dry lentils since they are split in half when dried. They don't need to be soaked before cooking. Lentils are high in protein, folacin, iron, zinc, thiamin, and fiber.

MILLET: A small, mild flavored seed that is similar to rice in texture and flavor. Use it in place of rice or in a "Millet Burger" (page 258.)

MISO: A naturally aged soybean paste used for adding flavor to soups, sauces, etc. Three types of miso found in the United States are red (made from rice and soybeans), hatcho (made from soybeans), and barley (made from barley and soybeans).

NUTRITIONAL YEAST: A common flavoring in vegetarian cooking. It is available in flakes or powder form and gives food a "cheesy" taste. Try it in soups, stews, and sauces or on popcorn. Some brands are good sources of vitamin B_{12}, but not all; check the label Don't confuse nutritional yeast with dry active yeast or brewer's yeast, which both taste terrible!

PINE NUTS: Also called piñola. Like other nuts, they are high in fat, so use sparingly. Try them roasted on salads.

QUINOA: A high-protein grain with a texture similar to barley. Rinse before cooking and use in place of rice, or in salads with beans and vegetables.

SEA VEGETABLES: Examples are nori, dulse, kombu, wakame, and arame. Agar is a substitute for gelatin.

SESAME OIL: A strong tasting oil used in Asian cooking. Because the flavor is so concentrated, just a few drops imparts a wonderful flavor to your cooking.

SOY SAUCE: An aged product made from soybeans and often wheat. Tamari is similar to soy sauce but it is made with little or no wheat. Soy sauce is very high in sodium, although lower sodium versions are available. Kikkoman Lite Soy Sauce contains 100 milligrams sodium per 1/2 teaspoon.

Storing Whole Foods

Hopefully, you are changing your buying habits to include more "whole" foods such as whole grains and beans. Keep the following in the refrigerator: whole grain flour, nuts, seeds and nut butters, tofu, whole grain breads, and baked goods.

The Best Fat-Free and Low-Fat Foods

Going through all the fat-free products now available could take months! That's why we were attracted to a new book from registered dietitian Elaine Moquette-Magee, called *Taste vs. Fat* (Chronimed Publishing, Minneapolis). The author and taste-testers nationwide rated the best and worst brand-name low-fat and fat-free foods. We've included highlights of their list to give you a start in selecting the best tasting products. Of course, there are more and more fat-free foods going on the market every day, so just because a food isn't listed here doesn't mean it's not good!

We have found that there is often a wide variety of reactions to low-fat and fat-free food, depending on personal preferences. When talking to clients and friends, though, it seems like the main brand names keep popping up: Healthy Choice, Entenmann's, and Snackwell's. Also, don't overlook the store brands (such as Safeway Enlighten) which are introducing new salad dressings, soup in a cup, etc. You may not agree with every rating here, but considering the opinions of others is better than trying every new product you see.

All the foods listed are either fat free or low fat. Here are the results, according to *Taste vs. Fat:*

BEST CRACKERS:
- Snackwell's Cracked Pepper Crackers/Reduced Fat Zesty Cheese/Fat Free Wheat Crackers
- Keebler Reduced Fat Club Crackers

BEST SNACK FOODS:
- ◆ Reduced Fat Lay's Potato Chips
- ◆ Pringles Right Crisps

BEST CANNED SOUPS/CHILIS:
- ◆ Healthy Choice New England Clam Chowder/Garden Vegetable
- ◆ Campbell's Healthy Request: New England Clam Chowder/Chicken Noodle
- ◆ Hormel Fat-Free Vegetarian Chili

BEST SALAD DRESSINGS:
- ◆ Hidden Valley: Light Original Ranch/Fat-Free Blue Cheese
- ◆ Kraft Free: Thousand Island/Italian

BEST YOGURT:
- ◆ Double Delights Bavarian Cream with Raspberry Topping
- ◆ Continental Non-Fat Lemon Yogurt
- ◆ Colombo Low-Fat Yogurt

BEST VEGETARIAN BURGERS:
- ◆ The Original Gardenburger
- ◆ Boca Burger

BEST PASTA SAUCE:
- ◆ Rao's Homemade Marinara
- ◆ Classico di Napoli

BEST COOKIES:
- ◆ Snackwell's Reduced Fat Mini Chocolate Chip Cookies
- ◆ Reduced Fat Chips Ahoy
- ◆ Elfin Delights Reduced Fat Vanilla Sandwich

Best "ice cream" product:
- ◆ Breyer's Light Vanilla
- ◆ Healthy Choice Special Creations Cherry Chocolate Chunk
- ◆ Ben & Jerry's Low-Fat Cherry Garcia

Questions You May Have About Fat-Free Food

Why is sugar often the first ingredient listed in fat-free cookies and cakes? When the fat is taken out, something must be added to keep the product moist. This is often sugar. If you are trying to stay away from sugar, look for Health Valley products, which are sweetened with fruit, or try making your own.

What are all those funny sounding ingredients in fat-free salad dressings and cheeses? When you take out the fat in those products, something must be added to give the texture and mouthfeel of fat. Though they sound like exotic chemicals, most are from plants and trees. Here are a few common ingredients:
- ◆ *Cellulose gum:* Added to cheese to keep it soft and smooth. Modified form of a substance found in plants.
- ◆ *Xanthan gum:* One of many gums that are added to cheese and salad dressing to thicken them. Made from corn syrup. Other gums are carob bean gum (from the locust tree) and gum acacia (from the acacia tree).
- ◆ *Carrageenan:* Used in salad dressings and even low-fat hamburger beef as a thickener and fat substitute. It is made from seaweed.

Can you eat too many fat-free products? Make sure you get your daily fill of grains, beans, fruits, and vegetables before eating fat-free products. Fat-free desserts are highly processed and loaded with sugar; easy to eat, but the calories add up!

98   **WHAT ABOUT OLESTRA (OLEAN™)?** Proctor and Gamble is test marketing Olean, its brand of fake fat. It is synthetic, has a consistency and texture of fat, and cannot be absorbed by the body. It has no taste of its own, but takes on the taste of other ingredients. Products made with olestra will have fewer calories. For example: peach pie today, 405 calories, with olestra, 252 calories. Chocolate ice cream today, 270 calories per half cup; with olestra, 110. Why not eat the whole thing?

Health experts worry about several side effects. If you eat more calories, weight may rise. Olestra grabs onto the fat soluble vitamins A, D, E, and K, so the FDA requires olestra to be fortified with these vitamins. However, the other fat soluble substances in food may be leached out of those eating large amounts of olestra. The "olestra leakage syndrome" was named after some volunteers found they had loose stools, bloating, cramps, and occasionally anal leakage.

Be careful with this fat replacer.

IS IT TRUE THAT MARGARINE CAN LOWER CHOLESTEROL? An extract from pine trees, sitostanol, was added to margarine. In a sample of over 1,500 people in Finland, the product (Benecol) lowered cholesterol an average of 10 percent. So far, Benecol is only available in Finland. (Reference 33)

CHAPTER SIX

EATING AWAY FROM HOME

"Home is where the heart is."

Fast Food

We probably don't need to tell you—we live in a fast-paced world. However, the hectic pace of our lives shouldn't be allowed to destroy our health! Just in case you are waiting for your life to slow down before starting a new way of eating—be realistic! You'll probably never find that perfect time where there is a lull in your schedule—unless it's that quiet time in the hospital after another heart attack!

There's a positive trend growing among the fast food giants. They are starting to offer healthy choices. However, sometimes the life of these menu items is short. The "Border Lite Menu" at Taco Bell has been discontinued except for a few items. The McLean Deluxe was also recently taken off the McDonald's menu. People often say they want healthy food, but don't follow through in ordering it. Make sure to give your local restaurants positive feedback if they offer healthy choices on the menu. If they don't, ask for it. If enough people ask, and there is a demand, restaurants will improve their menus. Already, there are healthy options at many fast food restaurants. You needn't give up on "grab and go" type meals—just choose more carefully and stay away from places that don't offer a healthy choice. Also, let

100   restaurants know that you are avoiding them until they have a low-fat vegetarian option on the menu.

Good Choices

BREAKFAST:
- ◆ Pancakes with syrup (skip the butter)
- ◆ Fat-free muffins (McDonald's), English muffin (ask for it dry) with jam (McDonald's)
- ◆ Bagel or toast with jam or honey
- ◆ Cereal and skim milk
- ◆ Egg Beaters—good with mushrooms, onions, and peppers (prepared without added fat)

LUNCH AND DINNER:
- ◆ Bean burrito or tostada without cheese or with fat-free cheese (ask for lettuce and tomato)

PRACTICAL POINTS TO PONDER

Fast Food Tips

- ◆ *Most fast-food restaurants have salads or salad bars but don't carry fat-free dressing—bring your own.*

- ◆ *Vegetarian items such as refried beans will still have added fat. Ask if lard is used and, if so, avoid them!*

- ◆ *If a food is called "vegetarian" don't order it automatically. Those foods often have more added fat than other foods. The Veggie Cheese Melt at Denny's has 39 grams of fat!*

- ◆ *The choices at many fast food outlets are limited and may not be a complete meal. Bring some fruit and other snacks to fill out the meal.*

- Tossed salad or salad bar
- Baked potato (Wendy's, Arby's, and Hardee's)
- Meatless burger (ask them to leave off the meat and add more tomato, lettuce, onion, pickle, and mustard)
- Vegetable soups (Arby's)
- A meal of side dishes—often served at chicken, BBQ, and fish restaurants: Rice, baked beans, green beans, carrots, mashed potatoes, salad, peas, corn
- Noodles or rice bowl—served at many fast food restaurants in California and Hawaii

DESSERTS:
- Fat-free frozen yogurt (Dairy Queen, TCBY, I Can't Believe It's Yogurt, and many others)
- Sorbet and ice (Baskin Robbins, Häagen-Dazs, and other ice cream stores)

Here are some specific fast food menus. All menus have 8 grams of fat or less.

ARBY'S
- Plain baked potato au jus
- Lumberjack mixed vegetable soup
- Side salad with lite Italian dressing

AU BON PAIN (has many good choices!)
- Split pea soup and hearth roll
- Vegetarian lentil soup and petit pain
- Vegetarian chili and onion bagel

BOSTON MARKET (Formerly Boston Chicken)
- Steamed vegetables or zucchini marinara
- New potatoes
- Fruit salad

CARL'S JR.
- ◆ Baked potato lite with salsa (hold the butter)
- ◆ Side salad
- ◆ Orange juice

CAPTAIN D'S
- ◆ White beans
- ◆ Seasoned green beans
- ◆ Rice
- ◆ Dinner salad with low-calorie Italian dressing
- ◆ Bread sticks (up to 4, no added butter or salt)

EL POLLO LOCO
- ◆ Vegetarian burrito
- ◆ Side salad with salsa
- ◆ Corn tortilla

GRANDY'S
- ◆ Baked beans
- ◆ Green beans
- ◆ Seasoned rice or corn
- ◆ Salad bar with fat-free dressing or vinegar

JACK IN THE BOX
- ◆ Teriyaki bowl (ask to omit the chicken and soy sauce and double the vegetables)

FOOD FOR THOUGHT

Follow Frank for Lunch:

Dr. Barry usually fits in a workout at the "Y" during lunch but still has time to fit in a quick healthy lunch. He goes to Wendy's and gets the baked potato bar, topping his potato with broccoli and salsa.

KFC

- ◆ Red beans and rice
- ◆ Garden rice
- ◆ Green beans
- ◆ Mean greens

KENNY ROGERS ROASTERS

- ◆ Corn on the cob
- ◆ Steamed vegetables
- ◆ Honey baked beans
- ◆ Side salad

LONG JOHN SILVER'S

- ◆ Rice pilaf
- ◆ Side salad with your own fat-free dressing
- ◆ Green beans
- ◆ Baked potato

MACHEEZMO MOUSE (caters to the health conscious)

- ◆ Vegetarian burrito dinner and vegetables; or
- ◆ Vegetarian taco dinner and mixed greens

RAX

- ◆ Cream of broccoli soup
- ◆ Coleslaw
- ◆ Pasta salad
- ◆ Refried beans
- ◆ Spanish rice
- ◆ Three bean salad
- ◆ Tortilla or taco shell

ROY ROGERS

- ◆ Plain baked potato with gravy
- ◆ Side salad
- ◆ Baked beans

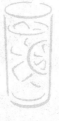

TACO BELL

- ◆ Bean burrito or bean tostada with fat-free cheese, fat-free sour cream, lettuce, and tomato. (These items are not on the menu; you must make a special request.)

WENDY'S

- ◆ Baked potato bar with steamed broccoli, tomato, and salsa
- ◆ Side salad with veggies, beans, and fresh fruit

WHATABURGER

- ◆ Potato with mushroom topping
- ◆ Garden salad with lite vinaigrette

ZU ZU'S

- ◆ Green salad with Salsa Rojo Epazote
- ◆ Veggie fajitas; or

- ◆ 2 black bean burritos without cheese
- ◆ Frozen yogurt

At the Salad Bar

TIPS:

- ◆ If you fill your plate up with only "rabbit food" you will be hungry an hour later! You also need to add some starchy foods like beans and corn, and have some bread or crackers and fruit.
- ◆ If you use "regular" salad dressing, you will turn a fat-free meal into a high-fat disaster. Bring your own fat-free dressing, or use vinegar or lemon or a low-fat dressing.

Depending on the restaurant, a salad bar can be a great place to eat a low-fat meatless meal.

Here's how the typical offerings on the salad bar rate.

GOOD CHOICES:

- ◆ Lettuce, spinach, radishes
- ◆ Broccoli, tomatoes, carrots, celery, corn
- ◆ Pasta salad (Most are surprisingly low in fat!)
- ◆ Three bean salad, kidney beans, garbanzo beans
- ◆ Any other vegetables, bean mixtures, or grain mixtures
- ◆ Canned or fresh fruits
- ◆ Jello salad

POOR CHOICES:

- ◆ Macaroni salad, potato salad, and other salads with mayonnaise
- ◆ Fried vegetables, fried Chinese noodles
- ◆ Cheese, ham
- ◆ Sunflower seeds and nuts (unless you use very little)
- ◆ Olives (unless you use very little)
- ◆ Pudding, mousse

Dining Out, Fat Free

OK. So now you understand the importance of fat-free dining to your health and well-being. You cook and eat fat-free at home. But what about dining out? The following story offers some suggestions to help you stay on course.

My brother-in-law Dave wanted to celebrate a family reunion. Being a very dedicated vegetarian, he knew the rest of the family members might feel deprived at a vegetarian only restaurant. But Dave was resourceful. Planning ahead, he was able to find his favorite food in a beautiful downtown San Francisco restaurant that also specialized in seafood.

The reunion came off without a hitch. Three generations ate to their heart's content. Those with special dietary needs were accommodated, and the others enjoyed the fresh seafood. Everyone left satisfied because the ambiance, presentation, color, taste, and amount were attended to. A great meal!

PRACTICAL POINTS TO PONDER

Ten Tips for Dining Out

1. *Call ahead to ask if the restaurant you are planning to visit has any vegetarian foods or can specially cook something up for you. Most nicer restaurants can easily do this.*
2. *When you are seated, ask the hostess that your server not bring the customary chips, crackers, biscuits, or other high-fat, pre-meal snacks. Also ask that they leave off the butter or margarine from the bread basket.*
3. *Have in mind what you will order when you get there. This will keep you from looking at the menu and being tempted.*
4. *If there is a shadow of a doubt about how a food is prepared or what ingredients it contains, ask! You may need to ask for a manager to get the correct information.*
5. *Ask in advance that all sauces, margarine, and sour cream be left off or served on the side. Also request that your toast or vegetables not be brushed with any margarine, oil, or butter.*
6. *If you are unhappy with the way the food is prepared— e.g., fried or a layer of oil on top—send it back! You are paying for your meal, and you should be happy with it.*
7. *Keep in mind that you are almost always getting more fat than you think you're getting when you eat out! Budget for it.*
8. *Bring with you anything that will help stay on track—fat-free dressing, package of butter buds, salt-free seasoning.*
9. *If you are ordering an alcoholic drink for your meal, have it with your meal, not before. Drinking on an empty stomach can increase your appetite and make it tougher to pass up the chips, bread, etc.*
10. *Most restaurants offer a dinner or garden salad. However, many add cheese, croutons, olives, nuts, etc., that increase its fat content. Ask about salad ingredients!*

TO AVOID FRUSTRATION If eating at a friend's home, explain your program ahead of time. Your friends will understand. Often, if you blame "this crazy meal plan" on your doctor (and I encourage you to, at least initially) an alternative can be planned. Better yet, offer to bring a delicious fat-free entree yourself!

Call ahead to the restaurant when eating out. Remember it's your money to spend wherever you choose. Most establishments will be eager to cater to your needs. Be very precise about your needs, however, and don't assume they know how to cook fat free.

TO AVOID EMBARRASSMENT Let everyone in your party know you are eating fat free. This will generate many interesting conversations about your choice, and is a good opportunity to *educate* your friends and be the center of conversation. However, make it clear this is your personal decision, and that your friends may eat whatever they choose.

At restaurants, check that menu choices fit your eating style. If not, call ahead and request a fat-free meal. If they cannot or will not provide one, suggest an alternate (better) restaurant to your friends.

TO AVOID TEMPTATION Pre-eat. That's right. If you know you will succumb, eat a meal or a snack at home. It will be easier to stick to the vegetables and bread if you are already full. But to endear yourself to the host, offer to bring a fat-free plate to the party. Not only will you help the hosts, but you will help yourself.

At restaurants, speak to the waiter immediately. Ask that the high-fat hors d'oeuvres and desserts not be placed in front of you.

FOOD FOR THOUGHT

Enjoy your dining experience—the presentation, amount, color, and taste. Don't forget the warm ambiance of friendly conversation and camaraderie! You will most likely enjoy your new eating style more than the old one, and I guarantee you will feel better when you leave the table.

If you already have scanned the menu, order even before being seated. Let waiters know you have special requirements and they usually go out of their way to please.

Common Restaurant Foods that are Fat-Free or Low-Fat

MEXICAN

TIPS:

+ Call ahead to see if the restaurant has any vegetables they can steam or grill for you, such as squash. If so, you can make your own vegetarian fajita; just skip the cheese, sour cream, and guacamole (or use tiny amounts).
+ Ask if the refried beans and rice are cooked with oil or lard. If so, find a restaurant that cooks with your health in mind. Ask if you can bring your own baked tortilla chips.
+ Ask the waitress to forego bringing the chips.

SUGGESTED MENU:

+ Gazpacho (cold vegetable soup) or jicama appetizer
+ Bean tostada (ask if the corn tortilla can be baked instead of fried) or vegetarian burrito topped with lettuce, tomato, peppers, and salsa
+ Mexican rice (if cooked without oil)
+ Steamed vegetables with salsa
+ Baked sopapilla with honey (ask them to bake instead of fry the sopapilla)

OTHER GOOD CHOICES:

+ Bean or vegetable stuffed enchilada
+ Steamed corn or flour tortillas
+ Bean tacos
+ Squash chili
+ Black bean soup

FAT-FREE ACCOMPANIMENTS: Salsa, lettuce, and tomato; jicama
salad, Tabasco

CHINESE
TIPS:

- ◆ Call ahead and find out if they can cook your meal without added oil.
- ◆ Find out what foods on the menu are fat free.
- ◆ If ordering a full meal that includes a high-fat egg roll or fried rice, ask what can be substituted for it.
- ◆ Dim sum is served on weekends at many Chinese restaurants. Carts are passed from table to table with small portions of many different foods. The ability to see a food before you eat it makes this a good choice.
- ◆ Tofu or bean curd is common in Asian cooking and can probably be substituted in any dish containing meat. Ask them to steam it instead of frying it.
- ◆ If you order noodles, make sure the noodles are soft and not fried or tossed with oil.

SUGGESTED MENUS:
- ◆ Bean curd soup
- ◆ Mixed vegetables with garlic sauce
- ◆ Won ton soup
- ◆ Vegetable lo mein (ask that it be prepared without oil or high-fat sauces)

- ◆ Steamed dumplings
- ◆ Bean curd with vegetables
- ◆ Steamed rice
- ◆ Hot tea and lichee sorbet

LOW-FAT ACCOMPANIMENTS: Chinese mustard, plum sauce, soy sauce (high sodium)

JAPANESE

TIPS:

- Steer clear of vegetable tempura (up to 56 grams of fat!) and see if you can have the vegetables steamed instead with the same dipping sauces.
- Japanese food tends to be lower in fat than some other oriental cooking. Leaving off the animal protein and extra oil should make most dishes fit your meal plan.

SUGGESTED MENU:

- Kinko no suimono (clear mushroom soup) or miso-shiru (miso soup)
- Maki (rolled and sliced rice sushi with cucumber)
- Soba noodles with bean sprouts, carrots, and tofu
- Japanese pancakes with sweet bean paste filling

OTHER GOOD CHOICES:

- Noodles or rice with any combination of vegetables

LOW-FAT ACCOMPANIMENTS: Wasabi (green horseradish), ginger-root, tempura sauce and soy sauce (both high in sodium)

THAI

TIPS:

- Thai food is often made with coconut milk, cream, or oil, so be sure to ask that those be omitted since they are very high in saturated fat.
- Many dishes are relatively low in fat—just ask that the meat be omitted.
- Vegetable dishes can be made lower in fat by omitting oil and fish sauce.

SUGGESTED MENU:

- Hot bamboo shoot salad
- Gaeng jued woon sen (vermicelli soup)

♦ Pahd puk (vegetables with sauce). Ask for coconut milk
and cream to be omitted.

♦ Thai salad rolls
♦ Fresh mango

FRENCH

TIPS:

♦ Though French cooking is known for using vast amounts
of butter and cream, the French are also known for eating
many vegetables and salads.
♦ You may be able to make a wonderful meal out of appetizers and side dishes.
♦ If unsure about sauces, ask for them to be left off or served
on the side.
♦ French bread is nearly fat free—enjoy!

SUGGESTED MENU:

♦ Mixed salad with red wine vinegar or steamed artichoke
with lemon
♦ Ratatouille Niçoise (eggplant, zucchini, tomatoes, and
garlic) or white beans with garlic and tomatoes
♦ Purée de pommes de terre à l'ail (potatoes mashed with
garlic)
♦ Fruit sorbet or bananas flambé (ask that butter be omitted
and orange juice or liqueur be used instead).

OTHER GOOD CHOICES:

♦ Steamed vegetables
♦ Plain pasta
♦ Puréed vegetables

ITALIAN

TIPS:

♦ Call ahead and find out if steamed vegetables and other
low-fat foods are available. Ask if any dishes such as mani-

cotti can be prepared with just vegetables.
- Bring your own fat-free salad dressing and butter buds for pasta.
- Ask which sauces are meatless and cheeseless.
- Ask for plain Italian bread instead of garlic bread. If bread sticks are served ask that they not brush them with butter or add cheese.

SUGGESTED MENUS:
- Tossed salad with red wine vinegar (or bring your own fat-free dressing)
- Baked ziti with marinara sauce
- Italian bread (no butter)
- Raspberry sorbet

- Tossed salad with lemon wedge or fat-free dressing
- Spaghetti with marinara sauce
- Steamed vegetables
- Capuccino with amaretto

- Lentil soup
- Pasta primavera without added fat
- Fresh fruit

- Tomato soup
- Fusilli with artichokes
- Latte made with skim milk, plain biscotti

INDIAN Indian food is mostly vegetarian but it is far from being fat free! With some education, some help from your waiter, and a bit of creativity in the kitchen, Indian food can be low fat!

SUGGESTED MENUS:
- Green salad with chutney
- Dahl with basmati rice

◆ Curried vegetables
◆ Peppermint tea

◆ Dholkas (steamed rice and bean cakes)
◆ Onion naan (roasted bread stuffed with onions and spices)
◆ Kachumbar salad (cucumber and tomato salad)

◆ Khasta rosti (roasted bread)
◆ Raita (yogurt and vegetables)
◆ Curried garbanzo beans
◆ Mazzo mango drink

The above information was compiled from *Simple, Lowfat and Vegetarian* by Suzanne Havala, M.S., R.D. © 1994, Vegetarian Resource Group. (Reference 34)

AT THE CAFETERIA

TIPS:

◆ Take a look at the whole cafeteria line before going through. That way, you can have your menu planned out.
◆ Cafeterias often add margarine to cooked vegetables; however, you can ask that all the juices be strained from your portion.
◆ Call ahead to see if your cafeteria carries any fat-free condiments—if not, bring your own. Also, ask how some of your favorite foods are prepared.
◆ There are usually several fruit salads that have no fat added.
◆ If you can't resist the temptation of seeing all the high-fat foods, you should stay away from cafeterias!

SUGGESTED MENUS:

◆ Strawberry and banana salad
◆ Steamed broccoli
◆ New potatoes
◆ Carrot coins

- Pinto beans
- Cornbread

- Fruited jello
- Frozen fruit salad
- Spinach
- Black-eyed peas
- Okra and tomatoes

- Three bean salad
- Spaghetti with marinara sauce
- Steamed zucchini and yellow squash
- Fresh fruit salad

PIZZA

TIPS:

- Order your pizza without cheese—for most people the crust is the best part anyway!
- Ask that they use no additional oil on the top or bottom.
- Top your pizza with all the veggies and sauce you desire!
- If you order your pizza delivered or get it "take out," you can add a bit of fat-free mozzarella or Parmesan cheese to it when you get home.

SUGGESTED TOPPINGS:

- Onions, peppers, mushrooms, artichoke hearts, roasted garlic, eggplant, spinach
- Tomato or extra tomato sauce
- Sliced olives (if put on sparingly)
- Capers (you can add this at home)
- Pineapple

ALL YOU CAN EAT BUFFETS Someone is cashing in on Americans' desire to get their money's worth when it comes to the dinner bill. If you have "eyes that are bigger than your stomach" at these places, you might want to choose a different sort of restaurant. I was pleasantly surprised to find that Old Country Buffet had two fat-free salad dressings to choose from and fat-free frozen yogurt for dessert.

GOOD CHOICES:
- ◆ Carrots
- ◆ Baked beans
- ◆ Corn
- ◆ Fruit salad
- ◆ Mashed potatoes
- ◆ Green beans
- ◆ Salad bar (see page 104)
- ◆ Rolls

STEAK HOUSES Most steak houses offer salads or a salad bar, baked potato, rice, and some type of fresh vegetables. Some offer a large salad bar extravaganza, which contains a lot more than just salad. A good low-fat meal can be had at a steak restaurant, especially one with a "food bar." However, first you must be able to pass up the steaks and all the fried foods available on the food bar. If you can't, it's safer to stick with restaurants with fewer temptations.

Best Bets—Chain Restaurants

All the following dinner menus contain 12 grams of fat or less. Dinner menus were chosen, assuming that most people eat a larger dinner.

APPLEBEE'S
- ◆ Steamed vegetable and salad plate (hold the cheese and bacon); bring your own dressing

BENNIGAN'S
- ◆ Steamed vegetable platter

- Baked potato
- Spinach side salad (hold the bacon and eggs)
- Bread (hold the butter)

CHILI'S This restaurant has a number of offerings for the heart-conscious eater; fat-free dressings, a low-fat vegetarian entree, some low-fat side dishes, and even fat-free frozen yogurt. You can have a tasty meal here.

- Side salad with no-fat honey mustard dressing
- Guiltless Veggie Pasta
- Southwest Sling Smoothie (nonfat vanilla yogurt, pineapple juice, orange juice, and strawberries)

BIG BOY RESTAURANT AND BAKE SHOP

- Vegetable stir-fry with rice
- Roll
- Fat-free frozen yogurt

CALIFORNIA PIZZA KITCHEN

- Grilled eggplant, Thai, or vegetarian pizza (all cheeseless)
- Field greens salad (bring own dressing)

DENNY'S

- Garden salad (bring own dressing)
- Split pea soup
- Plain baked potato
- Carrots and green beans
- Corn and peas
- Toasted bagel

OLIVE GARDEN

- Garden salad (bring own dressing or use vinegar)
- Minestrone soup
- Spaghetti with marinara sauce

RED LOBSTER

- Rice pilaf or baked potato
- Fresh vegetables (hold butter sauce)
- Dinner salad with lite Italian dressing
- Sherbet

RED ROBIN
- Meatless burger
- Side salad with fat-free dressing instead of french fries
- Steamer basket; vegetables and pasta with fat-free dressing

SHONEY'S
- Bean, tomato Florentine, or potato soup
- Grecian bread
- Salad bar with fat-free Italian dressing

SIZZLER
- Vegetable lasagna
- Salad with lite Italian dressing
- Minted Mediterranean fruit salad

SPAGHETTI WAREHOUSE
- Minestrone soup
- Spaghetti with marinara sauce

TGIFRIDAY'S On a recent "research trip" to Friday's, I was impressed with their offerings, including four vegetarian selections and two tasty fat-free dressings. For dessert, try a Fling—a fruit drink.
- Garden burger or Fresh vegetable baguette (hold the Swiss cheese)
- House salad (hold the garlic bread) with fat-free Italian herb dressing

Healthy Food in Any Language

Parlez-vous français? If you're a serious traveler, you may find yourself at the mercy of your waiter and pray that he speaks at least a little English. Here are a few phrases and words in French, Spanish, and German that will help you order heart healthy food!

FRENCH

I'm on a special low-fat (low-sodium) vegetarian diet.
Je suis un régime special sans matière grasse (sans sel), régime végétarien.
Please serve my food with sauces on the side and no added butter, oil, or cream.
Veuillez servir la sauce á côté dans une saucière, sans ajouter de beurre, d'huile, ou de crème.
Please serve my food without any sauce.
Veuillez servir ce plat sans sauce, s'il vous plaît.
No fried foods, please.
Pas de friture, s'il vous plaît.
Can I have this dish without the meat …chicken …fish …eggs …cream …butter …oil?
Puis-je avoir cette entrée sans viande …poulet …poisson …oeuf …crème …beurre …huile?
Do you have…
Avez-vous…
…skim milk?
…*du lait ecrémé?*
…fat-free or low-fat yogurt?
…*un yaourt sans matières grasses ou de régime?*
…steamed vegetables?
…*des légumes á la vapeure?*
…fresh fruit?
…*des fruits frais?*
…salad?
…*une salade?*

...a lemon wedge?
  ...une tranche de citron?
...fat-free salad dressing or vinegar?
  ...sauce salade sans matières grasses ou du vinaigre?
...plain pasta or rice with vegetables?
  ...des pattes ou riz natures avec légumes á la vapeure?
...hearty soup or stew without meat?
  ...un potage sans viande ou un ragoût sans viande?

SPANISH

I'm on a special low-fat (low-sodium) vegetarian diet.
  Estoy en una dieta vegeteriana baja en grasas (y baja en sodio).
Please serve my food with sauces on the side and no added butter, oil, or cream.
  Por favor sirvame mi comida con las salsas al lado y sin mantequilla, aceite, o crema.
Please serve my food without any sauce.
  Por favor sirvame mi comida sin salsa.
No fried foods, please.
  No alimentos fritos, por favor.
Can I have this dish without the meat ...chicken ...fish ...eggs ...cream ...butter ...oil?
  Puedo tener mi platillo sin carne ...pollo ...pescado ...huevo ...crema ...mantequilla ...aceite?
Do you have...
  Tiene...
...skim milk?
  ...leche descremada?
...fat-free or low-fat yogurt?
  ...yogurt simple o sin grassa?
...steamed vegetables?
  ...vegetales al vapor?
...fresh fruit?
  ...fruta fresca?

...salad?

...*ensalada?*

...a lemon wedge?

...*una rebanda de limon?*

...fat-free salad dressing or vinegar?

...*aderezo sin grassa o bajo en grasas o vinagre?*

...plain pasta or rice with vegetables?

...*pasta clara o arroz con vegetales?*

...hearty soup or stew without meat?

...*sopa abundante o estofado sin carne?*

GERMAN

I'm on a special low-fat (low-sodium) vegetarian diet.
Ich bin auf ein fettarme (salzarme) vegetarische Diät gesetzt.

Please serve my food with sauces on the side and no added butter, oil, or cream.
Bitte bringen Sie mein Essen ohne Butter, Öl, oder Sahne und die Sosse extra.

Please serve my food without any sauce.
Bitte bringen Sie mein Essen ohne Sossen.

No fried foods, please.
Nichts Gebratenes, bitte.

Can I have this dish without the meat ...chicken ...fish ...eggs ...cream ...butter ...oil?
Kann ich dieses Gericht ohne Fleisch ...Huhn ...Fisch ...Eier ...Sahne ...Butter ...Öl haben?

Do you have...
Haben Sie...

...skim milk?

...*Magermilch?*

...fat-free or low-fat yogurt?

...*fettloses oder fettarmes Joghurt?*

...steamed vegetables?

...*gedünstetes Gemüse?*

...fresh fruit?
  ...frische Früchte?
...salad?
  ...Salat?
...a lemon wedge?
  ...eine scheibe Zitrone?

PRACTICAL POINTS TO PONDER

Eating Right While Traveling

◆ *When flying, call the airline at least 24 hours in advance to order a low-fat vegetarian meal.*

◆ *Bring snacks such as pretzels, fresh fruit, and granola bars to fill in—airline food is getting mighty skimpy!*

◆ *Low-fat snacks available in most airports include fresh fruit, fat-free frozen yogurt, and bagels.*

◆ *Before making your hotel reservation, find out if healthy food choices are available at the hotel's restaurants. It's also wise to find a hotel that has a pool or fitness room.*

◆ *Reserve a hotel room with a refrigerator and/or cooking facilities. Having a refrigerator will allow you to have a fat-free breakfast in your room and healthy snacks for between meals.*

◆ *Try to go to a grocery store upon arrival to buy healthy foods. If staying with friends or relatives, this will ease the burden of them providing the foods you need or you eating foods out of guilt that you shouldn't.*

◆ *Dine at the chain restaurants mentioned in this chapter that you know will have healthy food choices.*

122 ...fat-free salad dressing or vinegar?

...fettloses oder fettarmes Salatsosse oder Essig?

...plain pasta or rice with vegetables?

...Nudeln (Teigwaren) ohne Sossen oder Reis mit Gemüse?

...hearty soup or stew without meat?

...füllende Suppe oder Eintopf ohne Fleisch?

CHAPTER SEVEN

WOMEN AND HEART DISEASE— THE WEAKER SEX?

"All's fair in love and war."

Heart disease and stroke are the leading causes of death among American women. Women are treated differently than men with heart disease. They have different risk profiles, develop the disease later in life, and have a different response to therapy. Women are in the unique position of having hormone decisions to make. And they are often not informed about the consequences of "estrogen replacement." Last year, over 485,000 women died from these preventable illnesses. I'd like to tell you about one of them.

My patient, Mrs. M, had just gone through the menopause. I was out of town when she rushed to the Emergency Department, complaining of weakness and difficulty breathing. An evaluation, including a complete pelvic exam showed anemia from vaginal bleeding. She was admitted to the Women's Pavilion of the hospital.

The next morning, I visited Mrs. M. "I feel lousy, like an elephant is sitting on my chest!" And she looked lousy—pale, sweating, gasping for air, she appeared very sick. A quick look through her chart showed only the anemia, now corrected with blood transfusions. No ECG had been performed to check the heart. No chest X-ray to check the lungs. No oxygen given for the breathing. Her heart wasn't even being monitored!

The "stat" ECG came as a shock. It clearly showed evidence of a major heart attack! By good fortune alone, she was stabilized in the coronary care unit with medical therapy. Although fluid filled her lungs, powerful water pills soon made her lose 10 pounds. Oxygen and digoxin helped boost the strength of the heart. However, extensive heart damage had been done.

The next day, after her heart catheterization showed blockages in all three main heart arteries and not amenable to bypass surgery, she asked me the inevitable question. "Why did this happen to me? I lost my husband last year. I'm getting ready to retire. I deserve a better fate!"

Of course, she was right. Feeling sick with anguish, I mulled over an answer. Mentally I reviewed her risk factors: former heavy smoker, overweight, lack of exercise, and the stress of losing her spouse. Although I didn't have an adequate answer, I stressed the future and hope for a recovery.

Several weeks later Mrs. M made an office visit. She was feeling better after cardiac rehabilitation but still wasn't her old self. "My daughter invited me to see Phantom of the Opera. *I very much want to go!" I knew the theatre steps were many and steep. However, after she passed her treadmill exercise test, I agreed she could go.*

I waited somewhat apprehensively for a call that weekend, but none came. Later in the week, she did call to say she had the best time ever, and no troubles at all! We were both very relieved.

It was a month later that the next call came. Mrs. M was found in her car, dead, by the side of the road. The coroner determined she had suffered a second heart attack, but was in enough control to get off the busy street and stop the car, saving other lives in the process.

Mrs. M taught me many lessons about women and heart disease, lessons I want to share with you now.

Is There Sex Bias in the Treatment of Heart Disease?

Certainly, there is no bias in Mother Nature. Slightly more women than men have heart disease, and more women than men die yearly from heart disease and stroke (485,000 a year). Heart disease and stroke are the leading causes of death in women.

For decades, medical research was an "old boy's club," run by men on male subjects only. The standard medical viewpoint was that heart disease was more prevalent in men. The proof? All the studies said so. When women were finally admitted into the research studies, the true extent of heart disease in women was discovered. Still the myths persisted.

More recently, research has shown further shocking disparities between the sexes. When men and women with chest pain were evaluated in emergency departments, twice as many men were admitted and received further evaluation and therapy. (Reference 35) A more recent review found that fewer, and often inadequate, diagnostic tests are performed on women suspected of having heart disease. Some differences were attributed to bias against emotional style. An emotional woman is perceived to have a far lower chance of heart disease than a woman with a businesslike affect. (Reference 36)

Even after sophisticated heart testing in men and women which was all positive for heart disease, men received further and more aggressive intervention than women. (Reference 37)

A higher proportion of first heart attacks are fatal in women, 8 percent more than in men. When "clot-busting" drugs are used to treat heart attack, striking differences in women are noted. They wait longer for the treatment to start. They have more complications, such as shock, heart failure, bleeding, and repeat heart attack. They have twice as many strokes as men (one of the most feared side effects of clot-busting drugs). Finally, the death rate is twice as high in women. (Reference 38) Additionally, women are several times more likely than men to die after bypass surgery.

It seems that men and women are evaluated and treated differently, even today. Controversy persists as to why, but there is general agreement that there is a bias.

Risk Factors

The factors causing heart disease are well known. Women share many of the same risk factors as men:

- ◆ Smoking
- ◆ High blood pressure
- ◆ High cholesterol
- ◆ Lack of exercise
- ◆ Stress
- ◆ Obesity

However, there are several persisting differences in women:

- ◆ More diabetes
- ◆ Higher triglycerides more important in the genesis of heart disease in women
- ◆ Higher incidence of congestive heart failure
- ◆ Dramatic increase in risk after the menopause
- ◆ "Atypical angina" more common than activity-related chest pain
- ◆ For those having a heart attack, a much worse prognosis, based on diffuse and severe coronary artery disease
- ◆ Greater risk of death after bypass surgery
- ◆ Greatly reduced risk if taking hormone replacement

THE MENOPAUSE No serious discussion of women's issues would be adequate without including the topic menopause. As the aging of America continues, women live nearly half their lives after going through the "change of life." This causes many effects, some of which are related to the absence of female hormones. The largest effect: increased cardiovascular disease and death.

Estrogen is one of the two principal female hormones, the other being progesterone. Estrogen is known to protect women from increased rates of heart disease after the menopause. In the huge *Nurses Health Study,* postmenopausal estrogen decreased the risk of heart disease by half. The good effects were evident even after adjustments were made for the other standard risk factors. (Reference 39) This has been recently reviewed and confirmed. (Reference 40)

Much of this protection is mediated through higher levels of HDL, the "good cholesterol" (Reference 41), as well as through other mechanisms. Users of estrogen after the menopause have lower rates of death (35 percent) from all causes than nonusers. However, those using the estrogen patch do not have beneficial effects on cholesterol. (Reference 42)

We now know that combined estrogen and progestin use also protects the heart. For those presently taking both hormones, their risk is only 39 percent of those not using hormones. This serves to reassure those women, who have not had a hysterectomy and take both hormones, that they do not lose any of the protective effect of estrogen alone. Both hormones are prescribed to reduce the incidence of endometrial cancer. (Reference 43)

THE FEAR FACTOR Other issues are raised when studying estrogen replacement. One that receives very little recognition or discussion is what I term "the fear factor." This is the notion that anything which could influence contracting "the big C" (cancer) is a fate worse than death. Many women, motivated by this fear, disregard or refuse therapy that could improve their health.

128　　　We already know that heart disease is the biggest killer of women. One in seven women 45 to 64 years old has some form of coronary heart disease. Over 485,000 women die a year. Compare that to all forms of cancer deaths in women, at 233,000. Estrogen reduces the risk of heart disease by half. The fear factor is an important consideration in the health and well-being of women. Let's examine the facts of estrogen replacement after the menopause. And let's do away with the myths.

OSTEOPOROSIS Hip fractures occur at a rate of 280,000 a year. Deaths from this disease approach 30,000 yearly.

Prevention includes improved diet, weight-bearing exercise, and smoking cessation. Additionally, estrogen therapy is very effective in preserving the strength of the bones after the menopause. The risk of hip fracture can be reduced by up to 60 percent (Reference 44).

Calcium is also important in the fight against osteoporosis. But how much do we need, how can we get it into our bones, and what are the best sources of the mineral?

A National Institutes of Health panel published guidelines on optimal levels of calcium, which vary with age and sex. See table below. (Reference 45)

OPTIMAL CALCIUM INTAKE	
GROUP	DAILY CALCIUM INTAKE (MG)
MEN:	
25-65 years	1000
Over 65 years	1500
WOMEN:	
25-50 years	1000
Over 50 years; Post-menopause:	
Taking estrogen	1000
Not on estrogen	1500
Over 65 years	1500

We all need calcium, but we also need vitamin D to absorb it. Vitamin D is available through sunlight, fortified foods, and supplements. Above 400 IU of vitamin D will suffice. For food sources of calcium, which are absorbed very efficiently, see table below.

After menopause, there is one very important thing you can do to build strong bones. Consider taking estrogen. At menopause, bone begins to lose calcium at a fast pace. The wrist and spine are affected the most. And age itself has the effect of slowing the pace of new bone growth. This affects the hips. Estrogen replacement has a major effect on retarding this bone loss.

Don't forget the beneficial effects of exercise on building strong bones. Weight-bearing exercise can build and preserve bone mass, thus preventing osteoporosis. In conjunction with estrogen and calcium, this is the most effective prevention program for osteoporosis.

CALCIUM SOURCES

FOOD ITEM	CALCIUM (MG)
Firm tofu (if made with calcium), raw, 1 cup	517
Tums	500
Yogurt, fat-free plain, 1 cup	452
Yogurt, fat-free vanilla, 1 cup	400
Collards, frozen, cooked, 1 cup	358
Tropicana orange juice plus calcium, 1 cup	333
Skim milk, 1 cup	302
Minute Maid enriched orange juice, 1 cup	293
Wonder enriched bread, 1 slice	290
Amaranth (grain), 1 cup	276
Turnip greens, frozen, cooked, 1 cup	250
Kale, 1 cup	180
Soybeans, 1 cup	176
Figs, 1/2 cup	143
Baked beans, 1 cup	139
Sherbet, 1 cup	103
Bok choy, 1/2 cup	79

ENDOMETRIAL CANCER Estrogen can cause cancer of the endometrium (lining of the uterus) when used alone. It causes about 5,900 deaths a year (Reference 46). If found early, endometrial cancer can be cured by having a hysterectomy (removing the uterus). Let's look at some statistics:

NUMBER OF ENDOMETRIAL CANCER CASES	
STUDY GROUP	**CANCER PER 100,000 PER YEAR**
Estrogen only users	390
No hormones	245
Estrogen+Progesterone	49
All groups combined	113

Using the combination of hormones dramatically decreases the risk of cancer of the endometrium. It also gives the added benefit of heart disease protection to a very susceptible population of women (Reference 47). If you have had a hysterectomy, you need only take estrogen.

BREAST CANCER No other cancer causes the fear factor in women like breast cancer. It is so common that most women have a friend or relative stricken with it. After the age of 50 or so, corresponding to menopause, the incidence rises dramatically. If all cases are included, even in 80 to 90 year old women dying of other causes, about 1 in 12 women will develop breast cancer. It is estimated that 145,000 new cases are found each year, and it causes 46,000 deaths a year. Most breast cancers occur at advanced age.

Breast cancer is the second most common cancer in women, after cancer of the lung. It is associated with a high-fat diet. There is no convincing evidence that breast cancer is caused by post-menopausal estrogen replacement (Reference 48). Several recent studies tend to confirm the little-to-no-risk effect of estrogen replacement. (Reference 49) There is controversy about premenopausal effects of estrogen on the development of breast cancer. For those with breast cancer, estrogen can stimulate its growth. There has been one study which seemed to indicate that, in women using estrogen at the time of diagnosis, breast cancer risk was higher. (Reference 50)

Realizing that risks for breast cancer vary, it seems prudent to sustain a low-fat meal plan to prevent this common disease. If you have very close family history (mother or sister with breast cancer) you can be tested for the breast cancer gene. You can discuss other ways to sustain your health, such as post-menopausal estrogen replacement, with your personal physician.

ESTROGEN REPLACEMENT THERAPY—WHAT TO DO? On balance, the numbers clearly indicate tremendous benefit with estrogen and progesterone use. Numbers, however, don't address "the fear factor." On this deeply personal level, several issues are important.

PRACTICAL POINTS TO PONDER

Take Charge of your Health Care

Reduce your risk factors for heart disease:
- *Stop smoking*
- *Eat right, cut out the fat*
- *Exercise regularly*
- *Check your blood pressure and cholesterol, and blood sugar. High sugar indicates diabetes*
- *If you have signs or symptoms of heart disease, such as chest pain, shortness of breath, fatigue, night sweats, or others, see your doctor immediately!*
- *After your examination, don't accept "it's all in your head" as an adequate explanation. Demand a full and careful inquiry into the cause of your symptoms. If your doctor balks, or doesn't treat disease if found, find another doctor!*
- *You can prevent and reverse heart disease! Make up your mind, and make the change!*

- During the prime of your life, from menopause to age 80, heart disease and associated deaths greatly outnumber breast cancer.
- The factors causing heart disease are well known, and many can be modified.
- The factors causing breast cancer are less well known, although fat in the diet and smoking can also be modified.
- Can you, as a woman, choose to die with heart disease rather than face the fear factor of breast cancer?
- Does the issue of osteoporosis (thin, fragile bones) influence your thinking? Estrogen and a low-fat, high calcium diet have been proven to prevent this disease of women.
- If you don't take estrogen, a low-fat diet, exercise, smoking cessation, and stress reduction can empower you to prevent both heart disease and cancer.

These issues are not easy. Please consult your personal physician for a detailed examination and discussion before deciding on hormone replacement.

CHAPTER EIGHT

SO WHAT'S STOPPING YOU?

"If you can't stand the heat, get out of the kitchen."
—Harry S Truman

Nothing will happen to your heart until you get stress under control. When you find out what you really value, it becomes easier to get there. This is the most important thing you can do for your heart: learn to reduce stress!

Stress, and How to Beat It!

A cardiac patient of mine, a rather young man to have a heart attack, decided to go through the Preventive Health Institute program after his recuperation. He did well, felt better, lost weight, and lowered his cholesterol and blood pressure. However, he kept complaining about the stress of his job. "I can't keep up with the demands," Joe said.

Six months later I saw Joe in the office. His face was bloated. His blood pressure was sky high, as was his cholesterol. He had gained weight. I asked him what happened.

"It's the job. It's killing me! I can't take the stress. I've even considered retiring, but I feel the others would think less of me as a person, like I was a quitter."

We discussed finances, pressure, health, and a host of other things. The issue was unresolved when he left. His biggest concern seemed to be the sense of failure he felt about quitting his job, as if he had to continue at all costs, no matter what the personal price.

We had spoken of priorities. Joe did take time to sit with his wife and make a list. It was emotional at times. Finally, they agreed on goals for the next several years.

One month later, Joe kept his scheduled appointment. As I walked in, he was smiling! "I'm retiring! And even though I have six months left, I feel like a weight has been lifted from my shoulders. I feel like a new man." He certainly was acting like a new man. He had beaten stress!

The very fortunate part of Joe's story is that, from then on, he found positive health changes much easier to accomplish. And I'm pleased to report Joe is a happy and healthy man today.

THIRTY-FIVE WAYS TO LEAVE YOUR STRESS (to the tune of "Fifty Ways to Leave Your Lover," by Paul Simon)
1. Take a walk in the rain.
2. Take a walk in the rain, holding hands.
3. Tried riding a bike lately? You never forget how.
4. Hike up your favorite hill.
5. Swim your troubles away.
6. Have sex often.
7. Join a group, any group.
8. Turn off the TV and find time to join a group.
9. Enjoy a good belly laugh.
10. Offer to help someone else more in need than you are.
11. Think positive.
12. Take control of your work stresses.

13. Be realistic. How bad is the worst thing you fear?
14. Live in the present. No one is good at seeing the future.
15. Bend a little, change a little. Perhaps a yoga class?
16. Stretch your neck and shoulders.
17. Learn a relaxation technique.
18. Listen to music you enjoy.
19. Practice deep breathing.
20. Take a break, even for 5 minutes.
21. Read a good book.
22. "Don't sweat the small stuff" because...
23. Everything is the small stuff.
24. Play Santa Claus this year.
25. Take a lunch break each day at work.
26. Learn to "problem solve."
27. Change a behavior that causes more worry than it helps.
28. Speak up. Others don't know if you are worried.
29. Pick up a hobby or sport that requires concentration.
30. Lower your shoulders once an hour to relax.
31. Explore your spiritual side.
32. Visit the church of your upbringing.
33. Invest 5 minutes a day daydreaming.
34. Take up a new sport.
35. Dance.

FOOD FOR THOUGHT

Stress Reduction Usually Comes Down To...

◆ *Exercise*
◆ *Getting connected with others*
◆ *Changing external causes of stress (like flex time instead of rigid hours)*
◆ *Self control (learn to will your body to relax)*

Your heart can't take the stress. Why?

I have a short story about my father. He was a smoker. A veteran of World War II, he worked for years at IBM. When it came time for me to graduate from Georgetown University, he had just finished a master's degree from New York University. Because of the stress of job, school, and the added financial pressure of a son headed to medical school, his heart attack came quickly and unexpectedly. The morning of graduation, he couldn't finish breakfast. The attack was fatal. He was 53. I believe stress did him in.

Some people are termed "hot reactors." They pay a high price for stress because their blood pressure rises to high levels, without their awareness. Over time, the heart suffers greatly. For example, volunteers compared physical stress on an exercise treadmill test with mental stress. The mental stresses were mental arithmetic, public speaking, reading aloud, and a timed tracing of an object in a mirror. During all the tests, they were given sensitive studies of the heart. In the 5-year study, the mental stress tests were twice as powerful in shutting down blood to the heart (ischemia). Those with ischemia due to mental stress had three times the risk of heart attack in the next 5 years! (Reference 51)

The good news: this bodily reaction can be unlearned. And this is fortuitous, because stress may be the single most important factor in recurring heart problems.

◆ A recent study (Reference 52) proved that mental stress constricted the coronary arteries as much or more than smoking and cocaine use!

◆ Another study (Reference 53) showed that men with high anxiety are six times more likely than calmer men to have sudden cardiac death.

◆ Depression in heart patients is a better predictor of future heart events than severity of heart damage, high cholesterol, and smoking (Reference 54).

The single most important problem we change at the Preventive Health Institute is not heart disease. It's the stress that led to the heart disease. It's the stress that blocks the changes necessary to get healthy.

Take the Life Event Test on page 139 and rate your stress level based on events over the past year. This may be the most important heart-related test you take! (Note: good stress and bad stress both affect you.) Then, when you identify your stress areas, it's the first step to changing to a healthier, less stressful lifestyle.

Anger

Anger is a common manifestation of depression, stress, or anxiety. Do you know someone who always seems to be angry? I'd like to tell you about Gene.

Gene was a "pain in the butt." Nothing was ever good enough. Nary a kind word passed his lips. The support group was fed up!

Don't ask me why, but at one group session, Gene raised his hand. "You people just don't understand. I saw it all in Vietnam! My buddies on the ground blown away. Some wounded so badly life wasn't worth living. Every time I hear the sound of a helicopter or plane, I duck and break out in a cold sweat. They won't get a chance to burn me ever again! I know, it makes me a terrible grouch, but I don't know any other way."

Did this outburst cure Gene's anger? Not a chance. However, after the group, another fellow befriended Gene. He, too, was a Vietnam War veteran, but had a slightly different perspective on life. They struck up a conversation, and quite a friendship.

The group noticed some subtle changes in Gene. The edges were still there, but perhaps not so sharp. Gene's explanation, which he shared with me months later—"I finally felt understood." He was less angry. He was also much more connected with people.

STEPS FOR CONTROLLING ANGER

- Stop and say to yourself, "I'm getting angry."
- Think about what will happen if you lose control. "If I lose control..."
- Ask yourself why you're really angry. "The real reason I'm angry is..."
- Reduce anger. "I need to cool down. I'm going to..."
- Reward yourself. "I did a good job. I'm going to..."

EXPRESSING ANGER

- Tell the person how you feel. "I'm angry!"
- Identify the specific event that made you feel that way. "I'm angry because..."
- Explain why you feel that way. "When you..., I feel angry."

Controlling Your Inner Self

Try the following relaxation techniques daily. The more you practice, the better it works. And, your new skill will be ready for you in times of increased stress.

Start under optimal conditions—a quiet comfortable room, where you will not be disturbed. As you improve your concentration, practice in other more public places. Before too long, you'll be able to practice self-control anywhere!

RELAXATION TECHNIQUES

- Interrupt your thoughts, stop thinking about your surroundings, and switch your thoughts to your breathing.

LIFE EVENT TEST

LIFE EVENT IN THE PAST YEAR	POINTS
Death of a spouse	100
Divorce	73
Marital separation	65
Jail term	63
Death of a close family member	63
Personal injury or illness	53
Marriage	50
Fired at work	47
Marital reconciliation	45
Retirement	45
Change in a family member's health	44
Pregnancy	40
Sex difficulties	39
Addition to family	39
Business readjustment	39
Change in financial state	38
Death of a close friend	37
Change to a different line of work	36
Change in number of marital arguments	35
Loan for a major purchase	31
Foreclosure	30
Kids leaving home	29
Trouble with in-laws	29
Outstanding personal achievement	28
Finishing school	26
Change in living conditions	25
Trouble with boss	23
Change in work hours	20
Change in residence	20
Change in schools	20
TOTAL SCORE	_____

YOUR SCORE:

300 OR GREATER: 80% chance of illness in the near future
150 TO 299: 50% chance of illness
LESS THAN 150: about 30% chance of illness

Reprinted with permission from Journal of Psychosomatic Research, *vol.11, pages 213-218, 1967, "The Social Readjustment Rating Scale," Elsevier Science Ltd., Pergamon Imprint, Oxford, England.*

Using your lower chest (the diaphragm) and your
stomach, take two deep breaths and exhale slowly.

♦ Scan yourself for tense or uncomfortable spots: forehead?
jaw? shoulders? Attempt to loosen this area up a little.
Allow your muscles to feel as heavy and warm as they can
in this amount of time. Body stress scanning usually lasts
two minutes but can be extended when you have the time.
People often do this when they must wait; while watching
TV, during traffic, or while in a line.

♦ Warm your hands momentarily.

♦ Do two quick yoga exercises:

> Rotate your head around in a circular motion once or
> twice.
>
> Roll your shoulders forward and backward a couple of
> times.

♦ Recall a pleasant thought, image, memory, or feeling just
for a few seconds.

♦ Take another deep breath from the diaphragm and return
to your activities.

♦ Quickly determine what it is about this situation, here and
now, that is annoying. (For example, the phone might be
ringing frequently, there may be excessive noise, etc.)

♦ Smile (outwardly or inwardly) and say to yourself,
"Leave my body out of this." This can either be aloud
or to yourself.

♦ Take two easy deep breaths. As you inhale count from 1 to
4, and as you exhale count from 1 to 4. As you exhale the
second breath, let your jaw go limp, and quickly spread
some of this relaxed, loose feeling to other tense muscle
groups.

♦ Resume your activities.

A short meditation is also helpful in controlling your inner
self.

♦ First scan your body, see what your muscles feel like,

attempt to relax and loosen up, and allow yourself to feel body sensations. Stay with this body scanning for a couple of minutes. Allow the muscles to feel as heavy and warm as possible. Focus on warmth in your arms and hands.

♦ Focus now on your thoughts. What are you thinking of? What kinds of thoughts have you had today, and which ones come to mind now? Are these upsetting thoughts or comforting ones? Dwell on the comforting or pleasant thoughts—place a greater emphasis on these thoughts.

♦ Focus now on your emotions or feelings. What do you feel? Content? Angry? Annoyed? Sad? Excited? Peaceful? Allow yourself to feel.

♦ Take three deep breaths (easy and slow) and return to your activities.

Practice these techniques daily!

Get on the Stick!

MOTIVATION Motivation is the inner drive that compels you to behave in a certain way. When you have motivation, you have (the tools for) it all!

The easiest patients I care for are the ones with large, built-in reserves of motivation. They are high-performance athletes even though they may not be in the Olympics or even participate in an organized sport. Injury or illness is seen by them as a temporary obstacle or barrier to their continued athletic performance. For instance:

♦ Three months of rehab? "I bet I can do it in two!"

♦ This is a very complicated disease? "Doctor, you tell me exactly what I need to do to get better, and I'll do it. I'm not your usual patient. I want to get well!"

What we know about motivation:

♦ Knowledge alone is not enough to motivate a long-term change in your behavior.

142

- Aversion technique can be somewhat helpful for some people. It is training the mind and body to be repelled by a negative addiction, such as smoking.
- Incentive technique can also be helpful. It works best at changing long term behaviors by rewarding something pleasurable after accomplishing positive behavior.
- Different types of motivation work for different people.

Seven Sure-Fire Ways to Improve Motivation!

Identify your core goals or desires, the things or actions or wants that only you know are most important to you. Core desires are genuine, clearly defined wants that cause you to be willing to put forth the effort necessary to make them become a reality. This even means overcoming seemingly insurmountable obstacles.

Core desires, Once you identify your core desires, they can motivate you to change your behavior from within. Your "coach" or physician can help you develop your core desires, but only you can have them.

DISCOVER YOUR OWN CORE DESIRES. For example: Being fit, if a priority, may bring you

...Physical attractiveness

...Love and laughter of friends

...Enhanced stamina

But how do you realize what these desires are? It starts with being honest with yourself. If you can get through the layers of excuses, explanations, and negative thoughts many of us have, you are on your way to being truly honest with yourself.

Recently, a visitor to the Preventive Health Institute had bypass surgery. Marty wanted to know what to do next: go back to the 80-hour-a-week job that he "really liked," or take early retirement and become the music coordinator at his church. When asked about his goals, out came a mish-mash of conflicting wants and needs. His life was a wreck! After an hour, we hashed out Marty's true goals. They included music, service to others, and a few more years of life to enjoy. He found his decision to give up the killer job much easier!

Then what? It will take an honest effort and a little time to brainstorm a short list of the really important things. We suggest sitting down with a spouse, friend, clergyman, or counselor to generate a short list. Give yourself an hour, and remember, it's not written in stone. Give yourself permission to go back and revise before settling on your true goals.

Bring Your Core Desire to the Surface with Daily Acknowledgment.

Unfortunately, if you don't think about your core desire often, it may slip from your grasp. With the hustle and bustle of daily life, we have plenty of thoughts crowding into our daily consciousness. Some suggestions for keeping the most important "up front":

...Post a message to yourself where you will see and read it daily

...Take a photograph of what you want the "new you" to look like and display it prominently. Alternatively, get a photograph of someone you respect or want to emulate and look at it often.

...Use the bathroom mirror to look yourself straight in the eye and affirm your new goals.

Actively Replace Old Beliefs with New Positive Ones.

For instance, replace "I've never been very physical" with "Exercise boosts my energy level!" Then go about restructuring your beliefs. Instead of "I'd rather die than walk in the rain," think about "Singing in the Rain" and how incredibly romantic it might be, with the right company.

Another example we hear frequently at the Preventive Health Institute revolves around food. "I could never live without meat" frequently becomes, "Most of the time, I feel better when I eat healthy food. I still like to splurge on the big holidays, however."

144

IDENTIFY THE OUTCOMES OF CORE DESIRES. This step can help to further define behaviors that can get you where you want to go. For example, if a global desire is better health, break it down into results: lower blood pressure, improved sleep patterns, increased energy, stress release, enhanced self-esteem, better sex life.

Try the traditional "I want to win the lottery." Then take it one step further. If indeed you had lots of money, what exactly would you do?

WHEN THE IMPULSE TO DROP OUT IS OVERWHELMING, SIMPLY DROP DOWN INSTEAD. Sticking to anything new is not easy over the long haul. There is a built in pessimism about trying again, perhaps a sense of failure. Realize your humanity! Life has its ebbs and flows. For example, it takes an average of three tries to stop smoking. We all know of someone who was successful!

Start again, by repeating the previous steps. Make sure your goals are realistic. After all, if you need hamburgers once a week rather than once a month, you are still a lot better off than twice a day! And you still have the option of reevaluating and changing again in the future. As we say at the Preventive Health Institute, "It's very hard to see the future."

BECOME AN EXCUSE BUSTER BY NOT MEETING THE EXCUSE HEAD ON, BUT BY SIDE STEPPING IT. For example, if you have started to believe "I hate driving to the gym," then tell yourself, "Nobody said I had to." Consider buying exercise equipment for home use. Try to reprogram yourself! Think differently. Avoid the negative by creating a positive thought or situation instead. Don't let a lapse become a permanent relapse!

DIFFERENT DRIVES FOR DIFFERENT LIVES, OR DIFFERENT STROKES FOR DIFFERENT FOLKS! Motivation is not necessarily born of logic, knowledge, or experience. It is locked within you, and you carry the key. Investigating what motivates you allows you to look at what triggers your behavior.

Why Do We Fail to Achieve Goals?????

◆ Most people start with impossible or unrealistic goals—"I want to lose 100 pounds." This is often seen in the sports world, where a young athlete may voice a desire to be in the Olympics. A trained coach, however, constantly tries to break success down into its components, for example, "Why don't you practice hitting the curve ball this week?"

◆ Striving to reach someone else's goal. For example, your spouse or parents.

◆ If the goal isn't really important to you—not your core desire—it's easy to sabotage the goal. You don't lose a thing!

◆ Little or no desire to achieve the goal. If it's easier to stay where you are, you will!

◆ Lack of self-awareness. So many of us don't know what we want out of life. It's easier to reach a place if you know where you're headed.

◆ Not measuring goals... what, how much, when. How will you gauge if you're improving? Batting average going up? Cholesterol dropping? Energy better? A's on the report card?

◆ Lack of visualization. If you don't know what the new, slim, trim, self-confident you will be like, you may be too afraid to make the change. Change often is scary.

◆ Lack of affirmation. "I am better or healthier or thinner today than I was yesterday." Say the words, repeat them, over and over.

◆ No reward system. "I lost those pounds, I deserve new clothes." If change isn't going to translate into something tangible in your life, why do it?

Stages of Change

Everyone goes through these stages, like a spiral, from one to the other, as the circumstances of our lives change. Try to pick out what stage you are in presently (Reference 55).

PRECONTEMPLATION: Not intending to change a behavior in the foreseeable future. You do not yet care enough about this behavior to consider change.

CONTEMPLATION: Intending to change a behavior in the foreseeable future (next 6 months, but not the immediate future). Good, at least you're thinking about it!

PREPARATION: Planning to change a behavior in the near future (next 30 days) and taking some steps toward change. Plan to do it during a low stress time.

ACTION: You have recently changed the behavior, or have tried and failed, but not given up. For example, quitting smoking usually takes two or three tries. Keep at it!

MAINTENANCE: Changed the behavior for more than six months. You succeed, one day at a time.

PRACTICAL POINTS TO PONDER

Motivation

- *Discover your core desire or goal.*
- *Acknowledge it daily.*
- *Think positive. The power of positive thinking is something that must be first believed, then you will see it!*
- *Where do you want to be for the rest of your life?*
- *Don't drop out, drop down.*
- *Side step excuses.*
- *Different strokes for different folks. What motivates you?*

Cheating

Here's a little story about food!

One of our participants at the Preventive Health Institute, let's call him Dan, was having a rough time. He had suffered two cardiac arrests and several heart attacks. After a new, experimental surgery, he had stabilized. He still struggled with his weight and cholesterol.

Dan was having a hard time with the concept of meat as a high-fat food. "I just love the smell of a barbecue. I rinse the hamburger, and dry it on paper towels. Then I partially cook it in a frying pan, and throw away the liquid fat. Finally, I broil it. Anything wrong with that?"

We spent several sessions in the group talking with Dan. People were very interested to know why he spent so much time and effort for one little burger.

It was several weeks later, when we were enjoying a dinner of nonmeat vegetarian burgers, buns, and all the toppings, that we found out. "This is great! Just what I enjoy. The smell, summertime, good conversation with friends. And these are a lot easier to make!" He later admitted he was just being stubborn, not wanting to admit the seriousness of his heart problems, and the burgers made him feel independent from his disease. Yes, once a month, Dan still needs a veggie burger on the grill. He has been able to make many daily, healthy changes without his independence feeling threatened!

Who Are You Cheating?

- ◆ Yourself, always. As you know, a treat or a feast on a special occasion "feels" different from cheating. It's that feeling that should alert you.

148

- ◆ Are you sometimes mad at the boss, and instead of telling the boss, you eat?
- ◆ Have there been stressful family interactions? A family member can be hard to confront. Do you take it out on food instead?

WHY ARE YOU CHEATING?

- ◆ Angry at someone? Stressed?
- ◆ No other reward system?
- ◆ Feeling self-destructive or depressed?
- ◆ Scorned or spurned?
- ◆ Lonely?
- ◆ Or, like Dan, having trouble accepting the reality of your present situation?

THE KEY TO THE PUZZLE: Why do you eat, why do you make harmful choices? Eating is much more symbolic than filling the belly and getting energy from food. Just look at our major holidays! The big event usually revolves around eating, and in the United States, overeating!

YOU CAN EAT MORE FOOD ON A LOW-FAT MEAL PLAN.

YOU CAN HELP YOUR EMOTIONAL STATE BY DEALING WITH IT, RATHER THAN SMOTHERING IT WITH FOOD!

Staying On Track

- *If you have heart disease and "cheat" often, you may need to examine stress, emotions, or purpose in life.*
- *If you are trying to be supportive to someone following the program, but cheat often, you may be undermining your loved one. This is termed "enabling" behavior.*

Other ways to avoid cheating:
- *Plan ahead. If you have plenty of low-fat, healthy food available, burgers and pizza will be less tempting.*
- *Drink lots of water.*
- *Exercise daily.*
- *Have plenty of snacks available. Use them.*

Healthy snacks to keep you from feeling like cheating (from a list compiled by participants in the Preventive Health Institute):
- *Fat-free cookies*
- *Fruit: raisins, apples, bananas, oranges*
- *Popcorn: a bushel full!*
- *Fat-free pretzels: Rold Gold, Mr. Phipps*
- *Angel food cake*
- *Fat-free frozen yogurt*
- *Vegetables: carrots, celery, cherry tomatoes*
- *Low-fat bread and honey or jam, or bagels*
- *Rice cakes: Quaker Oats*

We are all human and make mistakes. Let's try to minimize them. If we don't learn from our mistakes, we will be doomed to repeat them forever!

CHAPTER NINE

MOVE YOUR BODY

"If you don't move it, you lose it."

Some people with heart disease fear that exercise might hurt them. Exercise helps your heart and your mental attitude. Weight stays off with exercise. Bones stay strong. The best part is you needn't *work out* any more. Fitness is fun!

This chapter orients you to the new fitness. Find a program and a level that's best for you. Try cross training. And get the lowdown on exercise equipment.

Walking is practical for most people. It has the lowest dropout rate (among walkers, runners, bikers, and swimmers). It is very adaptable to conditions, it's portable, and it works! At 20 minutes a mile, 35 minutes of walking burns 150 calories. Up that to 2 miles in 30 minutes (or 15 minutes per mile) and you burn the same 150 calories and save 5 minutes!

For those with pain or foot, ankle, knee, and hip problems, consider the pool. Keep your head above water in a water aerobics class. Ex-runners may enjoy water running in the deep end, and burn 25 percent more calories than an equal time running on land. Lap swimming, for those who choose to keep moving, will burn the most calories. Enjoy that buoyant feeling, and improve fitness without pain!

As you get involved, consider wearing a heart rate monitor to get the feedback you need. Learn how good you feel after your program begins, and how to sustain that over time.

Rate Your Fitness Level

What type of activities have you done in the last month?

Yelling at the TV	0 points	_____
Walking	1 point	_____
Swim	2 points	_____
Work activity only	3 points	_____
Weight lifting	4 points	_____

How often did you exercise in the last month?

No exercise at all	0 points	_____
Once or twice	1 point	_____
Once or twice a week	2 points	_____
Three or more times a week	3 points	_____
Every day	4 points	_____

Do you hurt or ache after exercise?

Yes	0 points	_____
No	3 points	_____

How long do you exercise per session?

5 minutes or less	1 point	_____
5-15 minutes	2 points	_____
15-30 minutes	3 points	_____
More than 30 minutes	4 points	_____

What do you do in bad weather?

Skip exercise that day	0 points	_____
Walk in the mall	1 point	_____
Do calisthenics	2 points	_____
No change in home indoor routine	3 points	_____

SCORE YOURSELF:

0 to 5 points .... please start an exercise program!

6 to 15 points .... good start!

16 to 21 points .... great program!

Do you have any physical limitations to exercise?
◆ Arthritis of knee, hip, back
◆ Shortness of breath during exercise
◆ Chest pain with exercise
◆ Overweight causing inability to exercise

If you have any of the above conditions, be careful. You may want to consider pool exercise. Read the precautions and warnings section, page 169.

It's Time to Set Up Your Exercise Program!!!

It's best to accumulate 30 minutes of activity daily. Here's how. The Personal, Practical Program for New Athletes:
◆ Do something you like. If nothing comes to mind, try walking. Most people choose this because of the convenience.
◆ If you have physical problems, try pool therapy, water walking, water aerobics, or swimming.
◆ Go with a friend or join a group.
◆ Do it when you feel good. If mornings are your time, plan early exercise. If you are a night owl, afternoon or early evening might be better.

FOOD FOR THOUGHT

Did you know the Centers for Disease Control recommends a program of frequent moderate intensity exercise?.

A recent report by the Surgeon General on the benefits of physical activity agrees. One in four Americans don't do any exercise at all. The couch potato is at the highest risk of both heart attack and cancer. The report confirms that an accumulation of activity, adding up to 30 minutes most every day, enhances fitness and decreases heart disease, diabetes, colon cancer, and high blood pressure. (Reference 56)

- Have a little variety for bad days (both bad weather and bad mood days).
- You can form a habit faster by doing it most every day.
- Concentrate on aerobic exercise. Your heart, your mood and your schedule will benefit most from aerobic exercise.
- Start low and go slow. You can't get into shape all at once. It takes a while!
- Stretch after exercise. It relieves muscle soreness and gets rid of lactic acid buildup. It even relaxes the mind!
- Don't get discouraged! Fine wine takes time. Your youthful vigor will return. More to the point, you will be capable of performing like you did 10 to 15 years ago. (Yes, this includes sexual activity.)

About Exercise

Exercise is good for you! Remember the old saying "if you don't use it, you'll lose it?" It's true. Before you begin, listen to a little tale.

I'd like to take credit for motivating Maurice, but he came to see me without any prompting. Forty-five years old, he had a goal. He wanted to run the Pikes Peak Ascent race, held every August in Colorado Springs. This is no ordinary race. With an elevation gain of 8,000 feet, 14 mile distance, and variable climatic conditions, the faint of heart need not apply.

Maurice, it turned out, had made a New Year's resolution when we spoke in January. He had diabetes, high blood pressure, and high cholesterol, all mild. He was also 15 to 20 pounds overweight. After he passed his treadmill exercise test,

FOOD FOR THOUGHT

If you really want to find the time to exercise, unplug the TV. If you want to keep exercising, give away the TV.

the training began in earnest. He was smart. For a month he ran in a pool. Then as his stamina improved and the weather warmed, outdoor running commenced. Slowly and carefully, speed and distance increased.

I saw him several months later, to treat shin splints. At the same time, we checked his blood tests and weight, all of which had improved.

August came around, and I saw Maurice at the starting line. He waved and said he felt great! No, he didn't win, but I read his name in the paper. He had finished, and with a respectable time! Besides, he said, "The reasons for entering have nothing to do with winning."

Exercise Prescription

This is your checklist to prepare and plan your program.

WHY WILL YOU EXERCISE:
- ◆ improve appearance
- ◆ lose weight
- ◆ lower blood pressure
- ◆ improve energy
- ◆ reverse heart disease

WHEN WILL YOU EXERCISE: If you cannot decide when, it's unlikely you will start, much less stay with, your exercise. Pick a 30-minute period of the day, write it in your appointment book, and keep the appointment! Thirty minutes is 1/48th of the day.

TYPE: Should be aerobic, such as walking, jogging, biking, swimming, rowing, or aerobics class. Think about what you like to do. If nothing comes to mind, walk.

156

◆ Weight lifting and bodybuilding are not very aerobic.

◆ However, strength training is fine if you still have time after your aerobic exercise.

FREQUENCY: Should be five to six times a week. The benefits jump enormously from two workouts to three. On the other hand, exercising seven days increases the chance of injury.

INTENSITY: Should be moderate! No need to be a marathoner. Here are three ways to gauge this:

1. Target heart rate should be 65 to 85 percent of maximum. To calculate your maximum, take 220 minus your age. During exercise, take your pulse for 6 seconds and add a zero to find the beats per minute. See the table on page 158.

2. Perceived exertion, on a scale from "somewhat easy" to "very hard" should be in the moderate range, two or three steps up from "somewhat easy." See the chart on the following page.

3. If you cannot carry on a conversation, you are exercising too hard. If you don't even feel a little short of wind while talking, you may not be exercising hard enough.

If you have difficulty in gauging intensity, or if you find yourself exhausted afterward, consider wearing a heart rate monitor. This gives you instant feedback on how your heart is performing. You can then adjust to stay in your target heart rate zone. Polar makes a good one.

DURATION: Work up to 30 minutes of continuous activity. This duration is very dependent on the intensity of the activity. This does not include warm-up and cool-down.

PROGRESSION: As you exercise, feel better, and improve your stamina, you are encouraged to progress a little at a time. However,

only 10 percent progression per week is safe. For example, if you
choose to go 10 percent longer, don't also go 10 percent harder!

◆ Usually, people choose to speed up their activity level.

◆ For weight loss, you may need to exercise longer.

Prior to each session, prepare by dressing in loose, comfortable clothes and athletic shoes. A 5-minute period of gentle warm-up and light stretching is advisable. This will literally warm up the muscles, and make them pliant, and it will prepare the heart for exertion. This also cuts down the chance of injury; if you're injured, you can't exercise!

Following exercise, a period of slower activity should allow you to cool down. Stretch gently again. (The best stretching resource book is *Stretching*, by Bob Anderson.) This should leave you with the pleasant feelings of relaxation, calm, and well-being. Enjoy!

Monitoring Exercise Intensity

PERCEIVED EXERTION Use this chart to get in, and stay in, the moderate range:

1. Very, very easy
2. Very easy
3. Easy
4. Average or moderate
5. Hard
6. Very hard
7. Very, very hard

HEART RATE GUIDELINES These are only guidelines! Exercise up to the point you feel invigorated. Don't push it to the point of feeling bad. Consider a heart monitor if you are having difficulty. Polar makes an easy-to-use model.

HEART RATE GUIDELINES

AGE	65% OF MAXIMUM HEART RATE	75% OF MAXIMUM HEART RATE	85% OF MAXIMUM HEART RATE
35	120	139	157
40	117	135	153
45	114	131	149
50	111	128	145
55	107	124	140
60	104	120	136
65	101	116	132
70	98	112	128
75	94	109	123

Cross Training

To keep up interest, avoid boredom, exercise different muscles, and have a contingency plan for the weather, use cross training.

Cross training makes use of two or more different exercise methods to keep active. This also doubles your pleasure! Cross training can extend your activity level and duration. If you suffer from joint aches and pains, vary the joints you use (i.e., upper body and lower body) daily.

What are your goals? How fit do you want to be? Let's divide fitness into four broad categories. All will help your health. To reverse heart disease, you can plan on stepping up to the Health Improvement level.

◆ Yearning for Longevity—slow and low level
◆ Health Improvement—step up the pace of life
◆ Ready for Anything—need more variety
◆ Body Sculpting—lose lots of weight, keep it off, build muscles

Using cross training, I'd like to give specific examples of fitness programs you can use. I'll base them on the above categories of fitness you want to attain. If you're starting out as a

couch potato (sedentary), please just do a little until you find your
level of comfort.

LONGEVITY

- ◆ Move your body! Use a combination of activities.
- ◆ Monday, Wednesday, Friday take a 30-minute walk.
- ◆ Tuesday, Thursday, Saturday garden during the summer, ride a stationary bike during the bad weather.
- ◆ Sunday take the day off and relax.

Feel free to add in daily household chores, like climbing stairs, painting the house, moving boxes, etc., to your regimen.

If bone or joint pain inhibits you, consider water exercise. This consists of swimming, walking, or exercising in a pool, in water up to the armpits. Start with 20 minutes every other day, and work up to 30 minutes six days a week. This is the best non-weight-bearing exercise there is, and as such helps the heart and muscles without putting undue pressure on the bones.

As you grow in strength and endurance, consider the partial weight-bearing exercises such as biking and rowing, both indoor and outdoor. If you are up to it, you can add these occasionally to change your routine. Start at 20 minutes every other day, and build up to 30 minutes six days a week. Integrate these new activities slowly into your routine and enjoy the variety it brings to your life!

BENEFITS: This program has been proven to reduce risk of heart attack and cancer. Be prepared to wait a while until you see the benefits—they may not be evident till the latter stages of your life. At this level of exercise, you may not turn on the endorphins or feel like the athlete in you is coming out. Even though your muscles don't bulge, your heart benefits. The greatest amount of benefit is found if, instead of no exercise, you do a little something every day!

160   **HEALTH IMPROVEMENT** Let's focus on intensity. Use a heart monitor
or another method such as perceived exertion (page 155). Get
into the zone of moderate intensity for 20 to 30 minutes, five days
a week. The other two days, enjoy a relaxing walk.

To build intensity, many activities can be utilized. Brisk walking, hiking, biking, aerobics class or tapes, stair steppers, and
climbing machines will do. Singles tennis, racquetball, or handball
should work, but doubles probably will not. Consider wearing a
heart rate monitor to help you stay in your target heart rate zone
(that is, 65 to 85 percent of your predicted maximum heart rate).

It's true that the higher the intensity, the greater the fitness
and health benefit. But this is balanced by two things: injury
potential and fatigue.

There is a truism in sports science: if you are injured, you cannot exercise. However, using the cross training principle, try to
alternate more intense, weight-bearing days with less intense,
partial weight-bearing days. Thus some runners will run on alternate days, and swim or walk in between.

We have learned from athletes that, even when injured or
sick, most can swim to hasten recovery from accident, illness or
injury, without lowering their fitness level.

BENEFITS: At the Health Improvement level, you should notice
several quick results, as well as long-term benefits.

Almost immediately, you may feel more energy. Parameters
such as cholesterol, blood pressure, and heart rate may change.
Studies prove this level of fitness wards off infection and boosts
the function of the immune system. One of the best results at this
level is stress reduction. A calming of mind and muscle does
wonders for reducing levels of the stress hormones adrenaline
and cortisone.

Long-term, dramatic reductions in heart disease and cancer
rates are seen. The immune system boost may play a role in cancer reduction. HDL cholesterol levels rise to offset the buildup
in the arteries. A training effect is seen on heart rate: the greater

intensity over time, the lower the resting heart rate. Decline in lung function is lessened. Susceptibility to infection is reduced.

READY FOR ANYTHING At this level, you need a combination of intensity, duration, strength, and dedication.
- From 30 to 60 minutes of aerobic type exercise, five times a week.
- Intensity in the moderate range (60 percent of maximum).
- Resistance exercise, such as weight training or calisthenics, two times a week.
- Stretching to keep the joints smooth and capable of full range of motion.

Resistance exercise is used to build bone density, and strengthen and hypertrophy muscle. Far from the sweaty gyms of the past, there are many new and easier ways to get resistance exercise. (See equipment, page 163.)

This is the essence of cross training. Different muscles, alternating hard and easy days, combining endurance and flexibility.

BENEFITS: For those whose "athlete inside" is breaking out, the strength, flexibility, and endurance necessary to engage in vigorous sports is gained. Injury avoidance is another interesting advantage at the Ready for Anything level. This is true for young athletes as well as for the elderly trying to avoid hip fractures. Strength and balance training has been proven to reduce falls, which consequently reduces the chance of hip fracture.

The building of a slimmer, trimmer, stronger "all American" type of physique begins at this level. Along with the body comes an enhanced ability, sexually and in sports. Your "Golden Age Olympics" participants are in this group.

Lastly, along with the reduced risk of heart disease, enhanced functioning of the immune system has been demonstrated. There are fewer cancers at this level of fitness—just from exercise, without any other changes in food, stress, or other risk factors.

162   **BODY SCULPTING** Losing weight, and more important, keeping it off. Tightening and toning muscles and skin. A daunting task or an interesting challenge?

The longer and steadier the exercise duration, the longer the benefits last after the exercise ceases. Studies show that the increase in metabolism which occurs with exercise can extend 8, 10, even 12 hours afterward. So try to extend your walks to 45 minutes, or even an hour, three days a week. And in the spirit of cross training, add resistance training to build muscle—30 minutes twice a week. Add a swim to prevent stiffness and soreness, and take the seventh day off.

For water lovers, beware! Because fat floats, swimming may be deceptively easy. Monitor the heart rate to 80 percent of maximum (see page 158) during 45-minute sessions, six days a week.

For those with joint pain, consider biking three sessions and swimming three sessions weekly. Rest the seventh day. Resistance training can be utilized to maximize weight reduction.

BENEFITS: Long-term studies prove the only way to sustain weight loss is a daily exercise program. The easy part is losing weight, the hard part is keeping it off in the Body Sculpting level.

Increasing metabolism changes the energy balance. The faster the metabolism, the quicker the weight loss. As muscles grow, there is more mass to burn energy. (Our fat mass doesn't burn much energy.)

As you lose inches, the figure comes back. As weight drops, the joints feel better, as does the mood. Best of all, your risk of disease decreases—both heart disease and cancer.

Exercise Equipment

◆ Most exercise equipment, bought with the best intentions, collects dust sooner or later.

◆ Using exercise equipment tends to be boring. Try putting your equipment near a window, or in front of the TV, or have music nearby.

♦ Using exercise equipment can be isolating, lonely, and repetitious. There is less desire to cross train or enjoy the great outdoors if it's sitting in your home.

♦ All types of exercise equipment work—if you use them. Before spending the money, will you keep using them?

♦ The best equipment investment may be a pair of walking or cross training shoes!

Types of Equipment

TREADMILLS: For those who like to walk (or run) indoors. Fully weight-bearing exercise. Caution is indicated in those with leg, hip, or back problems.

Features available:
♦ Automatic or manual height adjustment
♦ Automatic speed regulator
♦ Computer programs, which vary from preprogrammed exercise to races and visuals

Types:
♦ Challenger 5.0
♦ Star Trac 2000
♦ Woodway
♦ Less expensive nonmotorized like Jane Fonda's or Bruce Jenner's

BICYCLES: Many types and brands, including:
♦ Outdoor: mountain and road
♦ Indoor stationary: LifeCycle, Cybex, Randal Windracer, Schwinn Air-Dyne
♦ Recumbent, perhaps better for those with back problems: Diamond Back HRT by Preference

They are all partial weight-bearing, resulting in less strain than walking. It is very important to be fit properly for comfort. Most bikes have seat, length, and bar adjustments. The most critical is seat height. With the leg straight and knee locked, the heel should touch the pedal. Then start to pedal with the ball of the foot, the knee slightly bent.

Accessories abound. Book holders, heart rate monitors, and pedal revolution counters are a few. Several can be equipped with video monitors to play specially edited bicycle races. Race along with the pros in the Alps!

◆ The Schwinn Air-Dyne can be used with both arms and legs, making for a hard session.

ROWING MACHINES: A great aerobic workout that emphasizes the upper body. Care must be taken with form, or the back can suffer. Non weight-bearing. Can be hard on the low back.

Types:

◆ Concept II Rowing Ergometer keeps track of speed, and distance, but doesn't visually catch the attention, thus can be boring.

◆ LifeRower is a little more visually pleasing, showing information on a computer screen.

STAIR STEPPERS: A great aerobic exercise. Very popular. A little less weight-bearing and less traumatic than running, which can be important for those with leg and back concerns.

Care must be taken to let the weight rest on the legs. There have been a variety of ailments attributed to leaning on the arms, elbows, and wrists in an effort to make the legs work faster.

Types:

◆ Stairmaster 4000 PT

◆ LifeStepper

CROSS COUNTRY MACHINE: Since these machines use both the arms and legs, the exercise can be very vigorous. They can be used with either arms or legs. There's no monitor or readout to hold your attention.

Types:
◆ Nordic Trak

RESISTANCE TRAINERS: The main emphasis for your heart should be aerobic exercise. Resistance training should be reserved for those with the time, energy, and desire to supplement their aerobic exercise with strength training.

FOOD FOR THOUGHT

A participant in the Preventive Health Institute, Danielle, had recently had a heart attack and angioplasty. She had, to her credit, also recently given up smoking!

Danielle was having a hard time with her exercise program. Never having been very active, she didn't know where to begin. And when she started walking with the group, she wheezed and was tired.

"What's wrong?" she asked during the second session. Laurin, our exercise expert, gathered enough information to conclude several things. First, Danielle didn't know how to gauge the intensity of her exercise. For her weight and level of fitness and smoking history, she was exercising too hard. After reviewing heart rate and perceived exertion, Danielle was able to settle into a more reasonable pace.

In addition, because of inactivity, deconditioning, and smoking, Danielle was suffering from exercise-induced asthma. Every time she exercised, she wheezed. A quick trip to her doctor for a check-up and an inhaler, and Danielle made rapid progress. "I feel so much better," Danielle told us. She had just finished a 30-minute walk, keeping up with the others without shortness of breath. "Thank you."

Types:

- Many types of free weights
- Rubber band resistance—Solo Flex
- Fixed weight machines—Universal or Nautilus
- Variable resistance pressure machines—Kaiser

HEART RATE MONITORS: An aid to keep you in your target heart rate and intensity zone. Many models are available.

Exercise for Fun and Profit

Benefits of aerobic exercise include:

- Decreased stress and weight
- Increased HDL cholesterol, increased energy and vigor
- Reduction of deaths (see page 171)
- Enjoyment of the freedom exercise brings to your heart and mind
- Reversal of heart disease!!!

You can even lower your blood pressure by aerobic exercise! (See table on the next page.) Over 140 adults, exercising three or four days a week for 10 to 37 weeks, were studied. Exercisers averaged reductions of 6 points diastolic and 7 points systolic. This meets or exceeds the effects of most drugs used for high blood pressure (Reference 57).

HOW MUCH WILL IT COST?

- 3,500 calories in 1 pound of fat
- Decrease calories by 230 a day for 7 days = 1,610 calories
- Walk 3 m.p.h. for 30 minutes = 315 calories for 7 days = 1,890 calories
- 1,610 calories + 1,890 calories = 1 pound of fat lost each week

PRECAUTIONS! 167

- *Chest pain:* Slow down and talk to your doctor. This symptom can go away in as little as two weeks on our program of moderate exercise, eating right, and stress reduction.
- *Dizziness during or after exercise:* Dizziness has different causes. Speak to your doctor. Don't exercise when dizzy.
- *Injury:* Substitute another form of exercise while recovering, e.g., swim instead of walk. Start slow and low, because an injured athlete cannot exercise effectively.
- *Hot weather:* Drink plenty of fluids (bring them with you), and exercise early in the day.
- *Cold weather:* Dress in layers, and cover everything, including fingers, ears, and nose. Consider exercising indoors. Go to an aerobics class or use your own tape on the VCR. Use a stationary bike, stair-stepper, rowing machine, or treadmill. Be sure to play music or watch TV to distract you from the surroundings!

MYTHS ABOUT EXERCISE:

- *"No pain, no gain."* Get real! Forget what the high school coach said. You should be able to appreciate the mental and physical relaxation of exercise without having to endure pain. If you do experience pain, something is

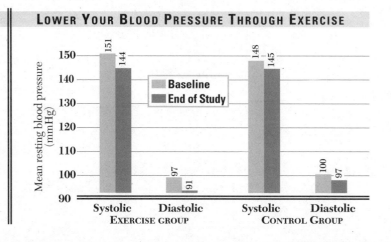

LOWER YOUR BLOOD PRESSURE THROUGH EXERCISE

Mean resting blood pressure (mmHg)

Baseline
End of Study

Exercise group: Systolic 151, 144; Diastolic 97, 91
Control Group: Systolic 148, 145; Diastolic 100, 97

168   wrong, and you should consult a professional.

♦ *"The harder the workout, the quicker the benefits."*
Especially for beginners, a hard session will cause pain, stiffness, and possible injury. For the heart, it's better to do a slower, sustained routine. Who said it had to be a *workout.* You don't have to run marathons to be an athlete. Perhaps you can call it "moving your body"!

♦ *"Sweating = weight loss."* Let's not confuse dehydration, which makes you feel terrible, with long-term weight (fat) loss. To prevent dehydration, always bring plenty of water. Drink every five minutes. If you wait till you feel thirsty, your body is already a quart low!

To accomplish long-term weight loss, long-term daily exercise is important. So don't get dehydrated! The best types of rhythms for weight loss are the longer, slower, moderate exertion sports. They are most efficient in burning fat, while relatively sparing the carbohydrate stores in the muscle and liver. Again, you don't have to run marathons to lose weight.

Warnings During Exercise

SERIOUS

♦ Abnormal heart action such as pulse becoming irregular; fluttering, jumping, or palpitations in chest or throat; sudden burst of rapid heartbeats; sudden very slow pulse when a moment before it had been on target.
Timing can be immediate or delayed.
Cause: Extrasystoles (extra heart beats), dropped heart beats, or disorders of cardiac rhythm. This may or may not be dangerous and should be checked out by a physician.

FOOD FOR THOUGHT

"The reasons for participating have nothing to do with winning."

Remedy: Consult your physician before resuming your exercise program. Medication may temporarily eliminate the problem and allow you to safely resume your exercise program; or you may have a completely harmless kind of cardiac rhythm disorder.

◆ Pain or pressure in the center of the chest or the arm or throat, precipitated by exercise or following exercise. Timing can be immediate or delayed.
Cause: Possible heart pain.
Remedy: Consult physician before resuming exercise program. Nitroglycerine may help.

◆ Dizziness, light-headedness, sudden uncoordination, confusion, cold sweat, pallor, blueness, or fainting. Timing is immediate.
Cause: Insufficient blood to the brain.
Remedy: Do not take the time to cool down. Stop exercising immediately and lie down with feet elevated, or put head down between legs until symptoms pass. Consult physician before next exercise.

LESS SERIOUS—SELF-ADMINISTERED REMEDIES

◆ Persistent rapid heart action near the target level even 5 to 10 minutes after exercise. Timing is immediate.
Cause: Exercise was probably too vigorous.
Remedy: Keep heart rate at lower end of target zone. Consider using a heart rate monitor to receive immediate feedback on your comfortable "target zone." This is between 50 and 65 percent of your predicted maximum heart rate. Drink fluids during exercise. If this does not help control the high recovery rate, consult physician.

◆ Flare-up of arthritis or gout that usually occurs in hips, knees, ankles, or big toe (weight-bearing joints). Timing can be immediate or delayed.
Cause: Can be trauma to joints that are particularly vulnerable.

Remedy: If you are familiar with how to quiet these flare-ups of your old joint condition, use your usual remedies. Rest and do not resume your exercise program until the condition subsides. Then resume exercise with these suggestions: lower level of intensity, protective footwear, softer surfaces, try swimming or water walking. If the joint problem is new, consult a physician.

Fitness and Longevity

Fitness is a powerful indicator of health and longevity. Dr. Stephen Blair, the president of the American College of Sports Medicine, did a series of fitness tests (stress tests) on 100,000 men at the Cooper Clinic. His astounding finding? When you are fit (as measured by minutes on the treadmill) your weight hardly matters. And thin, sedentary people? They have correspondingly higher levels of heart disease than those who remain fit. He feels the fitness level, not the weight, is the important factor in disease prevention. (Reference 58)

Figures 1 through figure 3 show age-adjusted death rates by physical fitness categories for all causes, for cardiovascular disease, and for cancer. Death rates show a striking decline across fitness categories in both men and women.

For all causes of death, death rates go down as fitness increases:

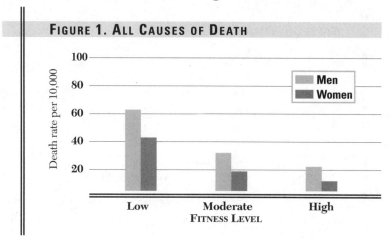

For cardiovascular deaths, death rates go down as fitness increases:

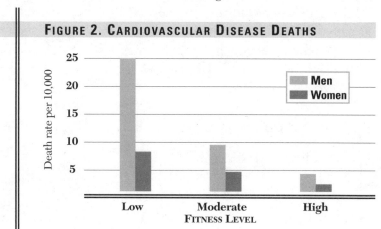

For cancer deaths, death rates go down as fitness increases:

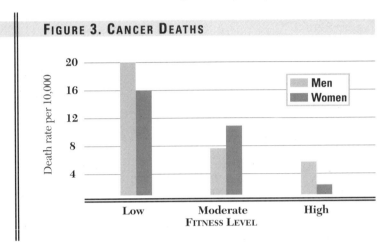

FIGURE 3. CANCER DEATHS

Figure 4 illustrates the relation between fitness and all-cause mortality in men with high levels of other risk factors. Men in the moderate fitness category have much lower death rates than the low-fit men in each other risk factor group.

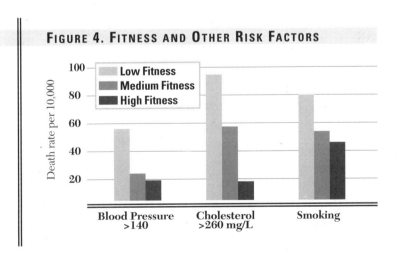

FIGURE 4. FITNESS AND OTHER RISK FACTORS

CHAPTER TEN

KICK THE HABIT

"Puff, the magic dragon, lives by the sea..."
—Peter, Paul, and Mary

Stop Smoking Program

Today is the first day of the rest of your life! How long you live and how you live is to a great extent controlled by you. Nothing changes unless you are ready and willing. We can empower you to change and make the process easier for you. We can save you money to boot!

Smoking negatively impacts your quality and quantity of life. It causes shortness of breath, emphysema, pneumonia, wheezing, and bronchitis. It causes more heart disease than lung disease! It causes impotence, bad breath, gum disease, sinus congestion, and ulcers. Worst of all, it harms your children and turns them into smokers.

Our program can help you! Even if you have smoked for most of your life, you can benefit from stopping. Think about it, and quit now! It is critical to prevent and reverse heart disease.

Think about why you smoke. It's important to know if you use smoking as a stress reducer (there are better stress reliefs), or if you are addicted (probably), or if you just have a bad habit. Once you know, there are many behavioral control strategies we can teach you.

Start the program by picking a quit day. This is the day you start to be a non-smoker. Sign a non-smoking contract! To help

174 break the old habit, pick up a new one! Exercise helps to keep the weight down and reduce stress, but any new habit will do, as long as you do it every day.

Medication is available to control the withdrawal. The nicotine patch, or nicotine gum, is available without a prescription. A drug called clonidine can help control cravings. Antidepressants can help insomnia. In higher doses, antidepressants can help the depression sometimes felt after smoking cessation. There is a high level of depression in heavy smokers! Anxiety medicine can help anxiety problems. These symptoms are common and short term. Ask your physician.

Weekly visits to your doctor are encouraged to monitor medication and your response. They also help bolster motivation and can help you overcome any difficult times. Stress reduction is important, so you're not tempted to take it out on yourself by smoking.

We can help you enjoy life and feel better. Go ahead, kick the habit!! Sign on with the program, to improve your lifestyle. Take the step today, and enjoy a better tomorrow.

DIRECT EXPENSE AT $1.50 PER PACK

PACKS A DAY	COST PER MONTH	COST PER YEAR
1	$45.00	$547.50
2	$90.00	$1,095.00
3	$135.00	$1,642.00

How Much Does Smoking Cost?

Research shows there are many indirect costs associated with smoking. Increased medical expense; lost wages due to illness; damaged clothing, furniture, carpeting, and drapes; and cleaning costs amount to about $1,500 a year.

Direct Expense per Year $_____ + $1,500 = $_____ Total

Could you find something else to spend the windfall on? How about a vacation? A new wardrobe?

Dispelling the Myths About Smoking

Take this test on smoking, based on some of the questions we've had at the Preventive Health Institute. True or False?

◆ *If you have smoked for a long time, it's not worth stopping now.*

FALSE. *Stopping now will immediately reduce your risk of heart and blood vessel disease. It also relieves shortness of breath and the tendency to catch infections of the sinuses and lungs.*

◆ *Most smokers don't want to quit.*

FALSE. *Most smokers want to quit. Research shows 65 percent of smokers would like to stop.*

◆ *Women now are smoking less.*

FALSE. *Although smoking in general has decreased, smoking among young females has increased.*

◆ *I can avoid getting fat when I quit smoking.*

TRUE. *Although you will have a tendency to put on a few pounds when you quit (3 to 6 pounds), you can counteract this. An exercise program helps. So do the products used to quit, nicotine patches and gum. And eating low-fat foods does a lot. If you do put on a few pounds, you are much better off than if you continue smoking.*

◆ *Older smokers find it easier to quit.*

TRUE. *Men break down nicotine faster than women. Women are more likely to stick with cessation groups. For either sex, relief of symptoms such as shortness of breath, cough, and chest pain make it easier to succeed at quitting!*

A Practical Program to Quit and Stay Quit

GET READY!

- Think about why you smoke.
- Think about how you would feel better if you quit.
- Before lighting up, ask if you really need this.
- Add up all the money you save if you quit.
- Cut down either the number of cigarettes or the number of times you smoke.

GET SET!

- Set a quit date.
- Sign a stop smoking contract. Give a copy to a loved one.
- Many smokers say cigarettes are their "friends." What or who are your *true* friends? Call or write them. Surround yourself with supportive non-smokers!
- Plan ahead. What will you do if you get the urge to smoke?
- Change your smoking routine. Do you smoke when you drink coffee? Switch to orange juice. Smoke after meals? Take a walk before clearing the table.
- When you go out, pick a smoke-free environment like a movie theatre or smoke-free restaurant. Avoid the temptation of a smoky bar.

GO!

- Get nicotine patches or gum at the pharmacy, and have them available everywhere—in the car, at work, in your purse or wallet.
- The night before your quit day, throw out your cigarettes, lighters, matches, and ashtrays.
- Buy sugar free candy, gum, and toothpicks. Put them where you used to keep your cigarettes.
- Dry clean your clothes.
- Take frequent walks around the block.

1. Prevent and reverse heart disease!
2. Stay away from places you used to smoke.
3. Delay when you have the urge—it will pass.
4. Take one day at a time.
5. Spend the money you save from smoking on a nice treat for yourself!
6. Enjoy a long, passionate kiss.
7. Take a hike. Besides enjoying the smell of the outdoors, your new-found lung capacity will take you places you only dreamed about before!
8. Have a discussion with another non-smoker about how good you feel.
9. Develop your (damaged) sense of smell. Put on a blindfold and identify 10 different smells. Then go to a floral shop and do the same.
10. Put all the money you are saving in a large glass jar. Count it every day.

The Smoke Test—How Dependent Are You?

If you have had a hard time quitting in the past, take this test to determine how dependent you are on smoking.

How soon after you awaken do you smoke your first cigarette?
Within 30 minutes	1 point	_____
After 30 minutes	0 points	_____

Do you find it difficult to refrain from smoking in places where it is forbidden (such as church, library, theatres, etc.)?
Yes	1 point	_____
No	0 points	_____

178   Which cigarette would you most hate to give up?
      The first one in the morning   1 point _____
      Any other   0 points _____

      How many cigarettes a day do you smoke?
      26 or more   2 points _____
      16-25   1 point _____
      15 or less   0 points _____

      Do you smoke more frequently during the first hours after awakening than during the rest of the day?
      Yes   1 point _____
      No   0 points _____

      Do you smoke even when you are so ill that you are in bed most of the day?
      Yes   1 point _____
      No   0 points _____

      What is the tar content of your brand?
      High   2 points _____
      Medium   1 point _____
      Low   0 points _____

      Do you inhale?
      Always   2 points _____
      Sometimes   1 point _____
      Never   0 points _____

                                            TOTAL: _____

SCORE
      0-6 .... low to moderate dependence
      7-11 .... high dependence
      (Reference 59)

You Can Quit Smoking

◆ *It takes an average of two to three tries for many people to quit for good. As my friend says, "Opportunity only knocks three or four times!" Keep trying!*

◆ *Only you will decide if you will be a non-smoker!*

◆ *Fool yourself. Chew toothpicks or sugar free hard candy. Take a walk. Bite your fingernails.*

◆ *The urge passes! Wait, and it will leave.*

◆ *Give up slavery to nicotine. Be free!*

◆ *If you have anxiety or depression, treat it in a more health-enhancing way.*

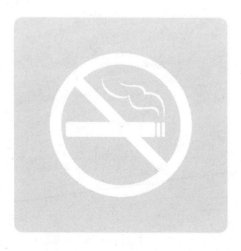

CHAPTER ELEVEN

SHOULD I BE TAKING A SUPPLEMENT?

"Just a spoon full of sugar helps the medicine go down"
—*Mary Poppins*

Wouldn't it be great! No need to prepare food, just touch the Starship Enterprise's food synthesizer, and out pops all you need for your health. Or backpacking trips made easy. All the nourishment in pill form. Very light. Easy to prepare. Quick.

Very futuristic. And perhaps science will take us there eventually. For the present, what our heart needs is whole food, not more pills. The right kind of food will help us reach our goals of good health, longevity, and prevention of disease like heart disease and cancer. The wrong kind will make us fat and get us sick.

Many people turn to vitamin and mineral supplements, hoping they are the keys to good health. It's true, vitamins and minerals—called micronutrients because they are needed in small amounts—are necessary to help your body perform its many functions. However, before you consider taking a supplement, read on to find out exactly what micronutrients are, how much you need, and the best way to get them.

Vitamins, Minerals, and Your Heart

In this section, we provide an overview about nutrients and specific functions for heart health. Foods listed as sources are only those recommended on the Healthy Heart Formula Food Plan.

RDAs (Recommended Dietary Allowances, 1989) are listed for men and women, age 51 or over. When one RDA is listed, it is the same for men and women.

Vitamins

VITAMIN A, its precursor is beta carotene

RDA 5,000 IU or 1,000 mcg. RE (microgram retinol equivalents), for men; for women, 4,000 IU or 800 mcg.RE

For practical purposes, beta carotene is recommended since too much vitamin A can be toxic.

As an antioxidant, dose of beta carotene is 25 mg. or 25,000 IU.

By eating plenty of fruits and vegetables, you should get all the beta carotene you need to prevent and reverse heart disease!

Recent studies confirm that whole foods rich in beta carotene, not supplements, prevent heart disease and cancer.

BETA CAROTENE SOURCES

FOOD ITEM	BETA CAROTENE (MG.)
Sweet potato, 1/2 cup mashed	8.8
Apricots, dried, 5	6.2
Peaches, dried, 5	6.2
Carrot, raw, 1	5.7
Spinach, cooked, 1/2 cup	5.0
Cantaloupe, 1 cup	4.8
Pumpkin, cooked, 1/2 cup	3.8
Squash, winter, 1/2 cup	2.9
Tomato paste, canned, 1/2 cup	2.2
Mango, 1 cup	2.1
Beet greens, 1/2 cup	1.8
Grapefruit, 1/2	1.6
Parsley, fresh, 1/2 cup	1.6
Pepper, red, 1 whole	1.6
Broccoli, cooked, 1/2 cup	1.0

THIAMIN OR VITAMIN B₁

RDA 1.2 mg. daily, for men; for women, 1.0 mg.

Used in nervous system tissue and in carbohydrate metabolism. The need for thiamin goes up with the amount of carbohydrate in the diet.

Sources: Brewer's yeast, wheat grain, whole grains and enriched cereals and breads, legumes, peas, potatoes, asparagus, green vegetables.

RIBOFLAVIN OR VITAMIN B₂

RDA 1.4 mg. daily, for men; for women, 1.2 mg.

Used in energy metabolism and helps convert the amino acid tryptophan to niacin.

Sources: Brewer's and baker's yeast, fortified breads and cereals, nonfat dairy products, legumes and peas, mushrooms, spinach, sweet potatoes.

NIACIN OR VITAMIN B₃

RDA 15 mg. daily, for men; for women, 13 mg., but when used to lower cholesterol, 1,000 to 2,000 mg. daily.

Niacin is involved in many body processes, including converting food into energy the body can use.

In high doses used for lowering cholesterol, it often causes flushing of the skin and can irritate the liver, making it necessary to monitor the liver through blood tests.

Niacin consumption should be medically supervised when taken at therapeutic high doses.

Sources: Fortified cereals, pastas and breads, whole grains and flour products, brown rice, legumes, peanuts, asparagus, green peas, corn, peaches, blackberries.

PANTOTHENIC ACID OR VITAMIN B₅

Estimated safe and adequate intake: 4 to 7 mg. daily

Releases energy from carbohydrate, fat, and protein.

Sources: Nonfat dairy products, white and sweet potatoes,

184   corn, legumes and peas, nuts, avocado, broccoli, whole
       grain cereals, mushrooms, tomatoes.

VITAMIN B₆ OR PYRIDOXINE

RDA 2 mg. daily, for men; for women, 1.6 mg.
Deficiency can contribute to high homocysteine levels,
    which increases heart disease risk when coupled with folic
    acid deficiency (Reference 60). Important in carbohydrate
    and protein metabolism and formation of hemoglobin.
Sources: Wheat germ, legumes and peas, cornmeal, quinoa,
    peanuts, walnuts, wheat bran, white and sweet potatoes,
    enriched cereals.

VITAMIN B₁₂ OR CYANOCOBALAMIN

RDA 2 mcg. daily
Deficiency may cause high homocysteine levels. Deficiency
    also causes pernicious anemia and nerve dysfunction.
    Needed for energy metabolism and to make blood cells.
Sources: Fortified cereal, egg whites and nonfat dairy prod-
    ucts. Spirulina, miso, and tempeh may list vitamin B₁₂ on
    the label but they may not be reliable sources.
Strict vegetarians may want to take a vitamin B₁₂ pill. Note
    that a microgram (mcg) is one millionth of a gram!

BIOTIN

Estimated safe and adequate intake: 30 to 100 mcg. daily
Used in the synthesis of fatty acids, and carbohydrate and
    protein metabolism. Important for the health of the circu-
    latory system.
Sources: Yeast, nuts, soy flour, whole grains, cauliflower,
    peas, vegetables.

VITAMIN C OR ASCORBIC ACID

RDA 60 mg. daily; when used as an antioxidant, 1,000 mg.
    daily

Helps vitamin E regenerate its antioxidant effect. Less vitamin E is necessary when vitamin C is available, to prevent heart disease. Other functions include wound healing, immune system function and folic acid metabolism. Also improves absorption of iron. Deficiency causes capillary fragility and scurvy.

Sources: Guava, citrus fruits, kiwi, mango, broccoli, melon, peppers, berries, tomatoes, cabbage, potatoes.

VITAMIN D OR CALCIFEROL

RDA 5 mcg. daily

Controls calcium metabolism. Important along with calcium in keeping bones strong after menopause.

Produced by the skin when exposed to sunlight and found in fortified milk. People living in northern areas (or those who stay indoors) may need a supplement during winter months if they don't drink fortified milk. The skin's production of vitamin D decreases with age.

VITAMIN E OR ALPHA TOCOPHEROL

RDA 10 mg. daily, for men; for women, 8 mg., when used as an antioxidant, 400 IU daily. (In a supplement, 1 mg. = 1 IU)

VITAMIN E CONTENT OF FOOD	
FOOD ITEM	VITAMIN E (IU)
Wheat germ oil, 1 Tbsp.	20.3
Sunflower seeds, 1 oz.	14.2
Almonds, 1 oz.	6.7
Cottonseed oil, 1 Tbsp.	4.8
Safflower oil, 1 Tbsp.	4.6
Wheat germ, 1/4 cup	4.1
Peanut butter, 2 Tbsp.	3.0
Mayonnaise, 1 Tbsp.	2.9
Peanuts, dried, 1 oz.	2.6
Mango, 1 medium	2.3

A supplement is suggested. Use the "dry" vitamin E to avoid excess oil. Proven to reduce coronary risk (Reference 61). Further studies show a 47 percent improvement in longevity, due to a 77 percent reduction in heart attacks. (Reference 62)

Vitamin E is often found in high-fat foods. Even if you did like wheat germ oil, the high levels of fat needed to get an antioxidant effect would be harmful. The influence of high vitamin E levels from food, on heart attack rates, is not clear. One study found no benefit from food (Reference 63), and the other found benefit only from vitamin E in food (Reference 64).

A supplement of 400 mg. of vitamin E daily is recommended at the Preventive Health Institute.

Folic Acid

RDA 200 mcg. daily, for men; for women, 180 mcg.

Used in cell production. Deficiency causes anemia.

Recent research shows that folic acid helps homocysteine levels stay normal to prevent atherosclerosis. There is speculation that the RDA should be raised to 400 mcg. daily. As many as two out of five elderly may not get enough (Reference 65). Aim for 400 mcg. daily from food sources. New information indicates a one and a half times higher risk of fatal heart attack in those with the lowest folate levels (Reference 66). The elderly, who because of poor dietary habits cannot get the 400 mcg. requirement, may want to take a folic acid supplement daily.

Sources: Legumes and peas, green leafy vegetables, asparagus, whole wheat and fortified cereals, oranges.

Vitamin K

RDA 80 mcg. daily, for men; for women, 65 mcg.

A fat soluble vitamin stored in the body; others are vitamins A, D, and E. Used by the liver to make the clotting proteins.

Sources: Kelp and seaweed, green tea, dark green leafy vegetables, broccoli, cauliflower, legumes, and peas.

Minerals

CALCIUM

RDA 800 mg. daily

Regulates muscle and nerve function. Important in the structure of bones. Especially important early in life, up to age 25, when the thickness of bones (bone density) builds the most. Calcium works especially well with weight-bearing exercise to build bone strength! Recent research shows supplemental calcium could reduce blood pressure in sensitive individuals. In women, estrogen allows the body to efficiently incorporate calcium into bone. Estrogen is recommended after the menopause to prevent osteoporosis.

See page 128 for calcium, dairy products, and suggested daily intake.

Sources: Nonfat dairy products, figs, green leafy vegetables, broccoli, molasses, legumes, almonds. Be careful to use only fat-free milk and dairy products. Excessive protein may harm more than help, causing a net loss of calcium.

CHROMIUM

Estimated safe and adequate intake: 50 to 200 mcg. daily.

A trace mineral that helps insulin work more efficiently. Low intake may be associated with high blood cholesterol levels and increased risk of heart disease (Reference 67). It is thought that many Americans have substandard intakes because of highly processed diets. Diabetics may benefit from a supplement or higher intake from food.

Sources: Brewer's yeast, whole grain foods, orange juice.

COPPER

Estimated safe and adequate intake: 1.5 to 3 mg. daily. Important in helping maintain healthy arteries, blood cells and blood vessels. Low intakes have been related to increased blood cholesterol in some studies. Also helps iron absorption (Reference 68).

Sources: Whole grain breads and cereals, nuts, dried beans and peas, dark green leafy vegetables.

IRON

RDA 10 mg. Iron is important in transporting oxygen throughout the bloodstream. Deficiency causes anemia, which is more common in premenopausal women and children. High levels could increase risk of heart disease, apparently by oxidizing LDL. Absorption of iron is inhibited by calcium in dairy products and supplements; also by tea and fiber.

Sources: Tofu, legumes and peas, dried fruit, molasses.

MANGANESE

Estimated safe and adequate intake: 2 to 5 mg. daily Assists in enzyme actions in body. Deficiency causes ringing in the ears and muscle weakness.

Sources: Whole grain breads and cereals, legumes, green leafy vegetables.

MAGNESIUM

RDA 350 mg. daily, for men; for women, 280 mg. Important for nerve function and muscle action, and may lower blood pressure. Implicated at deficiency levels in cardiac arrhythmias. Therefore, very important if the heart is stressed to have adequate levels.

Sources: Nuts, legumes, green leafy vegetables, whole grain cereals.

SELENIUM

RDA 70 mcg. daily, for men; for women, 55 mcg., as an aid to the antioxidant vitamins, up to 200 mcg. daily.

Some studies show low blood levels of selenium are related to increased risk of heart disease and some types of cancer.

Sources: Brazil nuts, cashews, kidney beans, mushrooms, onions. Also found in many vegetables, depending on how fertile the soil grown in is.

ZINC

RDA 15 mg. daily for men; for women, 12 mg.

Important for immune system function, wound healing, reproductive health, and taste buds. Deficiency causes inability to make sperm.

Sources: Wheat germ, miso, dried beans and peas, yeast.

PHYTOCHEMICALS Not artificial additives, but natural plant chemicals! There are thousands of these naturally occurring compounds in food which may not be in pills! Many are probably yet to be discovered. One reason to be careful with supplements: they may give you false assurance that your diet has all the nutrients it needs from a pill. However, if you don't eat whole foods in sufficient quantity, you miss out on all the benefits of phytochemicals. They are not available in pill form. The evidence is mounting that they are very useful to your health! Good health, cancer prevention, and low chance of heart disease come to those eating a fruit, vegetable, grain, and bean meal plan.

Here are just a few phytochemicals that we know about:

LIMONENE: (citrus fruits) Helps produce enzymes that may dispose of potential carcinogens.

ALLYL SULFIDES: (garlic, onions, leeks, and chives) Increase the production of glutathione S-transferase, which may make carcinogens easier to excrete.

DITHIOLTHIONES: (broccoli) Help form glutathione

S-transferase and may block carcinogens from damaging a cell's DNA. Yes, even though President Bush hated it, broccoli is good for you!

ELLAGIC ACID: (grapes, apples) Scavenges carcinogens and may prevent them from altering a cell's DNA.

PROTEASE INHIBITORS: (soybeans, dried beans) Suppress the production of enzymes in cancer cells, which may slow growth.

CAFFEIC ACID: (grapes and other fruits) Speeds the production of enzymes that make carcinogens more water soluble, which may aid in ridding them from the body.

FERULIC ACID: (fennel) Binds to nitrates in the stomach, which may prevent conversion to carcinogenic nitrosamines.

PHYTIC ACID: (grains) Binds to iron, which may prevent the release of "free radicals." These free radicals may oxidize LDL to form the "bad, bad cholesterol."

ISOTHIOCYANATES: (bok choy, broccoli, brussels sprouts, cabbage, cauliflower, collards, kale, kohlrabi, mustard greens, rutabaga, turnip greens, and turnips) Trigger the formation of glutathione S-transferase, which blocks carcinogens from damaging a cell's DNA.

INDOLES: (soy protein) Stimulate enzymes that make estrogen less effective, which could reduce the risk of breast cancer.

PHYTOSTEROLS: (soy) Slow down the reproduction of cells in the large intestine, which may prevent colon cancer (like high fiber content).

ISOFLAVONES: (soy) Block the entry of estrogen into cells, which may reduce the risk of breast or ovarian cancer. Pharmaceutical trials (Nolvodex) are underway to investigate this same mechanism to block breast cancer. May also lower cholesterol and increase HDL.

ARTIFICIAL COLORS AND PRESERVATIVES No known benefit (besides extending shelf life). Some may be harmful. Common reactions include:

- Allergy, as in asthma, hives, swelling, runny nose.
- Headaches
- Rashes

A partial list of additives: (There are many more!)
- BHT, BHA
- Monosodium glutamate (Accent)
- Salt (common table salt)
- Benzoates (sodium benzoate)
- Sulfiting agents (sodium metabisulfate used in restaurants)

PRACTICAL POINTS TO PONDER

Nutrients

- *Supplement vitamin E with 400 IU of "dry" E. Some selected groups may need extra vitamins. Special circumstances such as osteoporosis and anemia may require higher levels and a supplement.*

- *Remember the "new" heart disease risk factor—folic acid deficiency.*

- *Fruit, vegetables, and grains have natural chemicals, many of which are protective against disease!!!!!*

- *Mega dosing and supplements don't make up for a poor choice of foods (what you don't eat may hurt you)!*

- *Meat has a lot of harmful things in it! For your health, eat a lot more fruits, vegetables, whole grains, and legumes (beans and peas).*

◆ Tartrazine (FD&C Yellow No. 5)

◆ Antibiotics (found in meat and chicken)

◆ Hormones (found in beef)

◆ Nitrites and nitrates (found in hot dogs and lunch meats)

◆ Saccharin and aspartame (sweeteners)

For those of you wishing to minimize risk, organically grown food has the lowest levels of additives.

To keep the risks in perspective, however, please know that by eating more fruits and vegetables, you can lower your risk of heart disease and cancer. Washing produce well (or using products like FIT) can help if you worry about pesticides.

As we now know, by eating less meat, chicken, fish, and dairy we can also lower our risk of heart disease and cancer!

CHAPTER TWELVE

PHARMACEUTICALS

"Double, double, toil and trouble.
Fire burn and cauldron bubble."

—William Shakespeare
Macbeth

Drug Therapy

Read about Henry. He almost lost his life by disregarding his doctor's prescription. Then, his life was saved by the right drug at the right time. Help your doctor help you. Communicate with your doctor about whatever drug decision you make.

A patient of mine, Henry, was raking his yard. He started to suffer from excruciating chest pains. Rescue 911 was called, arrived quickly, and determined he was having a major heart attack! He was transported to the hospital.

The decision upon arrival quickly became whether to treat with a "clot-busting" drug to dissolve a blood clot blocking the artery saving heart muscle from damage. The risk of bleeding, especially of cerebral hemorrhage, was thought to be 3 or 4 percent. Henry's heart attack was very serious; it might very well be fatal. Of the several clot-busting drugs, he was given t-pa.

Henry had very good results. His potentially fatal heart attack was turned into a very small one. He went home in three days, feeling much improved. Good outcome, no side effects. It saved his life!

When he visited his cardiologist, Henry brought along a copy of his hospital bill. "Why does this t-pa cost so much? I think $1,200 a dose is excessive. Aren't there any alternatives?" As it turns out, Henry found that streptokinase is available for about 40 to 50 percent of the price of t-pa. For first time use, it works about as well. It has about the same rate of side effects as t-pa. And the experts are divided equally on the question of which drug is "better."

The makers of t-pa had just finished a major advertising campaign. National journals carried their ads, touting t-pa as superior, worth the money. And low and behold, sales went up. Coincidence, or change in usual practice based on sound scientific research?

Henry told his cardiologist, "If I ever again have to have a clot-busting drug, please use streptokinase. I don't have money to burn!"

Henry had been sensitized to this issue in the past. He had suffered side effects from two other heart drugs. He stopped one of them, without informing his doctor. He simply reduced the dose to reduce the side effects. Unfortunately for Henry, it was a bad move for his heart. Please don't repeat Henry's mistakes. Be courteous and inform your doctor. Form a team with your health care professional!

Factors in Drug Therapy

ADHERENCE Studies use the term "adherence" to describe how people take their prescriptions. Adherence drops the more frequently a drug is supposed to be taken. For example, many people don't take their medicine as prescribed:

◆ Prescribed daily: Taken 80 to 90% of the time
◆ Twice a day: 60 to 75%
◆ Three times a day: 40 to 50%
◆ Four times a day: 27 to 30%

Out of a ten-day antibiotic prescription, most people only take seven to eight days worth!

Drug taking also varies by the type of condition:

◆ Arthritis: 70%
◆ Epilepsy: 50%
◆ Diabetes: 50%
◆ Hypertension: 40%

COSTS Generic drugs usually cost 25 to 50 percent less than brand name or "proprietary" drugs. It's easy to spend $100 a month or more per drug. The drug companies want to recoup the expenses of research, development, and advertising. Generic companies don't have as much overhead. Generics are held to a slightly less strict standard by the FDA regulations. For a few drugs, such as certain types of digoxin and diuretics, this is a cause for concern.

"WHY AM I TAKING THIS DRUG?" Research shows that 60 percent of patients do not know why a particular medication has been prescribed. Please ask your doctor why you need this drug.

SIDE EFFECTS—I.E., BENEFIT VERSUS RISKS In most situations, the benefit is relatively small. A 50 percent reduction may mean a difference from 8 to 4 percent. In other situations, such as Henry with the heart attack, the benefits may be much greater.

Risks of drugs include allergy, nausea, fatigue, failure of the drug to work for the condition or disease, and drug interactions (with food or with other drugs).

As with everything in medicine, a detailed analysis of the risks versus benefits should be discussed prior to prescribing any therapy. Don't forget to ask about alternatives to the drug!

"I WANT TO DO IT ON MY OWN!" Some people, because of past experiences or anecdotal stories, are afraid or unwilling to take any drug. Others are unrealistic, in that they wish to be better, but will not make the necessary changes to ensure they will make themselves well.

"I FORGOT"—THE PASSIVE WAY TO REFUSE For any drug to have an effect, the patient has to believe in the need for the medication, and must take it as directed! Please, if you feel you cannot take a prescription for any reason, inform your physician!

A CAUTION ON DRUG INTERACTIONS For those on more than one drug, the possibility of interactions between drugs increases greatly. There may be:
- ◆ Failure of the drug to work
- ◆ Potentiation of the drug's action
- ◆ Diminution of the action
- ◆ Damage to liver, kidney, or other body system

WHY THE EMPHASIS ON DRUGS?
- ◆ Pharmaceutical manufacturers drive (i.e., fund) most research studies. As one of the largest multinational industries, the companies are constantly on the lookout for new products, and new uses for old ones.

  For example, the acne drug, Retin-A, was developed many years ago to treat teenage acne. Sales were moderate. It had a niche, however, and the company continued marketing. Several years ago, a research dermatologist studied its effects on age-related and sun-related wrinkling. After publication of the findings, the general news media picked up the story. Soon sales of Retin-A skyrocketed! Profits surpassed all records, mostly because the price went up as the popularity rose.

◆ Drugs are profitable.

◆ Pharmacology is taught in medical school.

◆ It is the tradition of many physicians to treat the disease, not the person (don't assign blame). The idea of personal responsibility for health is not stressed in medical schools.

◆ It's easier to take a pill than to make lifestyle changes. Taking a pill doesn't require much effort, and requires no change in habits. It takes less time to prescribe a pill than to explain the importance of exercise.

◆ People are not aware of the power they possess through diet, exercise, and stress reduction to influence their disease. They feel helpless against the disease and the medical system. They feel loss of control in their daily lives.

Waste and Duplication in the Industry

"Me-too" drugs start as useful, big-selling drugs for one company. Then, other companies come up with similar drugs, designed for the same condition, and promote heavily, hoping for a "big winner."

Prices vary, sometimes tremendously, within each class. Efficacy, or usefulness, can also vary, but to a much smaller degree.

CARDIOVASCULAR DRUGS:

◆ Anti-hypertensives, over 40 types
◆ Cholesterol lowering: Mevacor and Zocor (same company), Pravachol, Lescol
◆ Diuretics or water pills

ANTIDEPRESSANTS:
- ◆ Prozac
- ◆ Zoloft
- ◆ Paxil
- ◆ Effexor
- ◆ Serzone

ANTIBIOTICS:
- ◆ Cephalosporins
First generation – Cefalexin
Second generation – Cefactor
Third generation – Cefuroxime

What Will Companies Do to Sell the Product?

David Kessler, M.D., head of the Food and Drug Administration, recently commented on competition in the drug industry (Reference 69).

- ◆ Too many "me-too" drugs are developed and marketed.
- ◆ Companies put on "seeding trials" which appear to serve no scientific purpose. They pay doctors to prescribe their drug.
- ◆ Promotional materials may use false and misleading claims of superiority over a competing drug.
- ◆ Many companies, health insurance agencies, and agents try to get patients switched from their original prescriptions to "me-too" drugs marketed by their companies.

ARMACEUTICALS

Helping Medications Help You

Form an alliance with your doctor. Let your doctor help you be well.

If you don't intend to take a medication, tell your doctor. Hopefully, you will be ready to start the lifestyle changes necessary to make yourself well.

If you are having side effects, tell your doctor.

Ask if there are alternatives that are less expensive, and have fewer side effects, than the treatment being prescribed.

Don't take anything unless you understand what it is for and what it is supposed to do.

If you take more than one drug, make sure they don't interact with each other. Ask your physician under what conditions you should take the drug:

◆ *Full or empty stomach*
◆ *Time of day*
◆ *Mixed with or apart from other drugs*
◆ *Precautions such as sunlight exposure*
◆ *How long to take the drug*
◆ *What to do about side effects*

There is more than one way to achieve your goals. If you have questions or reservations, work with the experts to make a suitable plan!

CHAPTER THIRTEEN

A WORD ON CANCER PREVENTION

"A life lived in fear is a life half-lived."

You are trying to concentrate on reversing heart disease. This chapter explains the added benefit in cancer prevention you receive from the same lifestyle changes.

The fear factor affects many of us, like it did "Miss Nancy," a teacher. She was paralyzed by the fear of cancer, even after she noted the blood in the toilet.

"It's just hemorrhoids!" she said when I explained I needed to take a look. It was an epic conversation, extending not only through that visit, but through two months. Finally, she consented to the examination, which showed colon cancer. She wanted surgery to "get it out, all out." She didn't want to hear the surgeon talk about possible spread to the liver.

By great good fortune, "Miss Nancy" had a localized cancer, cured by surgery. She is alive and well today. She tries to stay that way with exercise, healthy food, and stress reduction.

National Cancer Institute News

SMOKING CONTRIBUTES TO CANCERS OF:

lung	mouth	larynx
esophagus	pancreas	bladder
kidney	stomach	uterus and cervix

35 PERCENT OF CANCERS ARE RELATED TO WHAT WE EAT. These cancers include:

colon	breast	prostate
stomach	liver	ovary
lining of the uterus (endometrium)		

AMERICANS EAT TOO MUCH FAT. Populations with a high-fat diet have a high incidence of colon, breast, and prostate cancer.

ALCOHOL Heavy drinking (over 2 drinks of alcohol per day) is associated with cancers of the:

mouth	throat	esophagus
liver		

The Case for Lifestyle and Cancer Prevention

There are four lifestyle elements that are associated with reduced cancer risk. By following the Healthy Heart Formula Eating Plan, you will automatically improve most of these areas. Remember the four F's:

FAT INTAKE: A high fat intake is generally related to higher cancer risk. Also, several studies have linked saturated fat intake with higher risk for lung and breast cancer. (Reference 70) Recent research proves older women can reduce their risk of lymphoma. Over 35,000 women were studied. A high meat diet and a high intake of fat from animal sources is associated with doubling the risk of non-Hodgkin lymphoma (a type of cancer). A decreased risk (only 64 percent of usual) is found with high fruit consumption. (Reference 71) Our program automatically cuts the fat and saturated fat in your diet to safer levels!

FIBER INTAKE: Insoluble fiber, the type found in whole grains and cereals, fruits, and vegetables, is associated with a decreased risk in cancer rates, especially of the colon. Recommended fiber intake is 20 to 30 grams per day. (The average intake in the United States is 5 to 10 grams.) See the following table.

FIBER CONTENT OF FOODS

FOOD	GRAMS OF FIBER
All bran cereal, 1/4 cup	10 to 13
Figs, 3	7
Wheat bran, 1/4 cup	7
Spinach, 1/2 cup drained	6
Blackberries or raspberries, 1/2 cup	5
Corn, 1/2 cup	5
Raisin bran, 3/4 cup	5
Prunes, 3	5
Broccoli, 1/2 cup	4
Dates, 5	4
Pear with skin, 1	4
Sweet or white potato, 1/2 cup	4
Whole artichoke	4
Bulgur, 1/2 cup	3
Orange, 1	3

PHYTOCHEMICALS: *("fi-toe-chemicals")* Vegetarians are generally healthier than their meat-eating counterparts for several reasons. Their diets are lower in fat, animal protein, saturated fat, and cholesterol, but their diets are also chock-full of whole grains, fruits, and vegetables.

Research shows that people who eat more fruits and vegetables have a reduced cancer risk. Why? Phytochemicals or plant chemicals in food are biologically active. Beta carotene is just one of many compounds, called carotenoids, that may be helpful in cancer prevention. Presently, there is only one way to get these compounds in your diet—by eating lots of fruits, vegetables, whole grains, and beans. There is a lengthier discussion of phytochemicals in chapter 4.

FITNESS: People who are more fit have much reduced rates of cancer. See below and Reference 58.

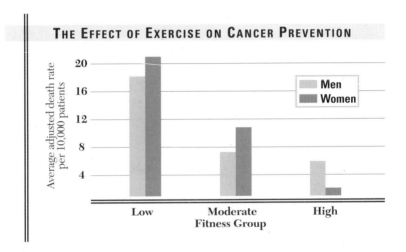

Case by Case Cancer Prevention
Cancer is the second leading cause of death in the United States.

LUNG CANCER is the most common cancer among both sexes, and the leading cancer causing death. Men have 94,400 deaths per year; women have 64,300. Clearly, women have caught up to men in lung cancer deaths, due in large part to intense advertising by the tobacco industry.
PREVENTION: Do not smoke. Quit now if you do smoke. (Chapter 10)

In women, **BREAST CANCER** is number two in deaths.
PREVENTION: Since breast cancer has been linked to a high-fat diet, cut way down on fat (Reference 72). There is some evidence that an eating plan high in antioxidants, especially beta carotene, also prevents this cancer. (See page 182.)

In men, **PROSTATE CANCER** is number two, with 41,400 deaths per year. It has been said that if you live long enough, you will develop prostate cancer.
PREVENTION: Since prostate cancer has been linked to a high-fat diet, cut down on fat (Reference 73).

COLON CANCER is next on the death list for both sexes. Men have 22,700 deaths per year, and women have 23,700.
PREVENTION: Since colon cancer has been linked to a high-fat, low-fiber diet, cut down on fat. In addition, those on a high-fiber diet have a reduced colon cancer risk. Take at least 25 to 30 grams of fiber every day to reduce cancer risk (Reference 74).

These four cancers—lung, breast, prostate, and colon—account for the vast majority of cancer deaths. (Source: *CA a Cancer Journal for Clinicians*, 1996, vol. 46, no. 1, p. 9) They can all potentially be prevented. You cannot change your genes, but you can control your habits.

Disproving Cancer Myths

Today is your lucky day! The day we disprove myths and misconceptions surrounding cancer, such as: "Doesn't everything cause cancer?" and "There is nothing I can do to reduce my risk."

♦ *All the techniques used to prevent and reverse heart disease will help prevent cancer!*

♦ *The leading cause of cancer is smoking.*

♦ *The next leading cause of cancer is SAD, the Standard American Diet.*

♦ *Other important causes are heavy alcohol use and sunlight.*

♦ *The fear factor is present in us all. Don't let it paralyze you! The facts and statistics tell us that cancer is a preventable, treatable, and in many cases a curable disease.*

CHAPTER FOURTEEN

DELIGHTFUL, DELICIOUS, DELECTABLE RECIPES

What You Will Find

◆ Breakfast Ideas (this page)
◆ Lunches On the Go (page 208)
◆ Fifteen-Minute Meals (page 209)
◆ A Month of Dinner Menus (page 212)
◆ Recipes (page 217)

Breakfast Ideas

◆ Low-fat pancakes with fresh berries
◆ Fat-free cereal with skim milk, yogurt, or soy milk, toast and juice
◆ Egg Beater omelette with mushrooms, green pepper, and fat-free cheese
◆ Toasted bagel with fat-free cream cheese, jam and cappucino
◆ Very Berry Shake (page 281), raisin toast
◆ Zucchini Bread (page 225) with fat-free cream cheese, fresh melon
◆ Pumpkin Muffins (page 222), oatmeal with cinnamon sugar
◆ Toasted fat-free pound cake with strawberries, hot cocoa

◆ Cereal with skim milk, fresh fruit, toast
◆ Grape nuts cooked in microwave with skim milk and dates
◆ Low-fat waffles with strawberry fat-free cream cheese spread and berries
◆ Fat-free yogurt with fat-free granola, cantaloupe, toast
◆ Crepes (page 251) with fresh peaches, latté with skim milk

Lunches On the Go

Listed below are some good choices for two favorite quick meals—frozen meals and cups of soup. Of course, leftovers also make good quick lunches as do sandwiches made of bean spreads, leftover tofu loaf or veggie burgers.

FROZEN MEALS: Please keep in mind that these meals are made for people trying to lose weight—most are 200 to 300 calories. This is not enough for an entire meal for most people! Add fresh fruit, salad, some type of bread, and skim milk or yogurt, and dessert if desired.

The following meatless meals have 6 grams of fat or less. Sodium is enclosed in brackets:

LEAN CUISINE:
◆ Macaroni and Cheese with Broccoli [460 mg.]
◆ Angel Hair Pasta with Vegetables and Marinara Sauce [420 mg.]

WEIGHT WATCHER'S:
◆ Garden Lasagna [540 mg.]
◆ Fettucini Alfredo with Broccoli [540 mg.]

SMART ONES:
◆ Lasagna Florentine [590 mg.]
◆ Ravioli Florentine [420 mg.]

CELENTANO'S:
 ◆ Broccoli Stuffed Shells [520 mg.]

HEALTHY CHOICE:
 ◆ Garden Potato Casserole [520 mg.]
 ◆ Macaroni and Cheese [580 mg.]
 ◆ Pasta Shells Marinara [390 mg.]
 ◆ Cheese Ravioli Parmigiana [290 mg.]

MICHELINA'S:
 ◆ Spaghetti Marinara [680 mg.]

LOW-FAT CUP-OF-SOUPS—THE NEW RAGE FOR A QUICK MEAL: Add a salad, fruit, and crackers and you've got a tasty, filling, high fiber meal!

Varieties that have 1.5 grams of fat or less and less than 500 milligrams sodium include: Taste Adventure Minestrone, Casbah La Fiesta, Nile Spice Lentil Home Style, Nile Spice Chili n' Beans, Fantastic Foods Jumpin' Black Bean, Fantastic Foods Leapin' Lentil Over Couscous, Fantastic Foods Splittin' Peas, Spice Hunter Kasbah Curry, and Nile Spice Red Beans and Rice. (Source: Supermarket Savvy Fact Sheet, © 1994, Leni Reed Associates)

Fifteen-Minute Meals

Some of these menus incorporate recipes from this book—page numbers are in parentheses; others use frozen or convenience foods.
 ◆ Tossed salad
 ◆ Pasta e Fagiol (page 261)
 ◆ Fresh fruit

 ◆ Broccoli coleslaw
 ◆ Sloppy Joes (page 263)
 ◆ Fresh mango or canned peaches

- Tomatoes in balsamic vinegar
- Tortillas with steamed vegetables and Dijon Sauce (page 240)
- Yogurt with strawberries

- Fiesta Pasta Salad (page 233)
- Baked tortilla chips with fat-free bean dip
- Fresh fruit salad

- Green Giant Create a Meal, sweet and sour vegetables cooked with tofu
- Vanilla pudding

- Health Valley fat-free chilli
- Tossed salad with fat-free cheese
- Frozen banana with fig bars

- Hash browns (found near eggs) with Roasted Red Pepper Sauce (page 243)
- Steamed frozen vegetable mix
- Bush's vegetarian baked beans
- Fat-free cookies and skim milk

- Leftover Pasta With Quick Alfredo Sauce (page 262)
- Steamed vegetables
- Sorbet

- Bean and Rice Burritos (page 245)
- Jello with fruit

- Minute Minestrone (page 229)
- Boursin Cheese Spread (page 217) on crusty french bread
- Fresh apple

◆ White kidney beans, cucumber, tomato, lettuce, sprouts, and green onions in fat-free vinaigrette inside pita bread
◆ Very Berry Shake (page 281)

◆ Hoppin' John (page 257)
◆ Coleslaw with fat-free ranch dressing
◆ Fat-free cookies

◆ Veggie burger on bun with sautéed onions and mushrooms
◆ Hash browns
◆ Fresh melon

◆ Tomatoes and cucumbers in fat-free vinaigrette
◆ Black bean tostadas (canned fat-free refried beans on baked corn tortilla)
◆ Healthy Choice low-fat ice cream

◆ Three bean salad
◆ Bulgur and Veggie Mix (page 270)
◆ Frozen yogurt with blueberries

◆ Instant couscous with chick peas, mixed vegetables, and Curry Sauce (page 239)
◆ Pita bread
◆ Microwave baked apple

◆ Tossed salad
◆ Pita pizza (pita bread topped with fat-free cheese, pizza sauce, veggies)
◆ Mango sorbet

◆ Fresh carrots and broccoli with fat-free dip
◆ Creamy spinach burritos (see Delightful Spinach, page 271)
◆ Mixed fruit salad

- ◆ Green Giant Create a Meal vegetable lo mein with tofu or black beans
- ◆ Berries and fat-free pound Cake

- ◆ Grilled vegetables (eggplant, squash, onions) on french bread with marinara sauce or fat-free cream cheese
- ◆ Fat-free hot fudge sundae

A Month of Dinner Menus

- ◆ Baby salad mix
- ◆ Spring Vegetables in Cream Sauce over angel hair pasta (page 265)
- ◆ Fresh fruit, cookies
- ◆ French bread

- ◆ Oriental Salad (page 235)
- ◆ Broccoli and Tofu Stir-Fry (page 248)
- ◆ Steamed rice
- ◆ Fruit sorbet

- ◆ Black Bean and Corn Salad (page 232)
- ◆ Greek Pilaf (page 272)
- ◆ Delightful Spinach (page 271)
- ◆ Melon balls

- ◆ Coleslaw with fat-free slaw dressing
- ◆ Boston Baked Beans (page 247)
- ◆ Bulgur and Veggie Mix (page 270)
- ◆ Healthy Choice Cookies n' Cream low-fat ice cream

- ◆ Leek and Potato Soup (page 227)
- ◆ Happy Family Dinner (page 255)
- ◆ Angel food cake with fresh fruit and 2 Tbsp. Cool Whip Free

◆ Romaine lettuce salad
◆ Ratatouille (page 274) with bow tie pasta
◆ Strawberry sorbet

◆ Grated Celery Root in Vinaigrette (page 238)
◆ Lentil Soup (page 228) garnished with tomatoes and fat-free sour cream
◆ Crusty sourdough bread
◆ Tiramisu (page 279)

◆ Raw vegetables with fat-free dip
◆ Baked tortilla chips with fat-free salsa
◆ Colorado Stuffed Peppers (page 250)
◆ Easy Blueberry Cobbler (page 278)

◆ Jicama and Orange Salad (page 234)
◆ Oat Nut Burgers (page 260) on wheat buns with all the trimmings
◆ Oven Fried Potatoes (page 273)
◆ Fat-free vanilla pudding with bananas

◆ Grated Carrots with Fat-Free Vinaigrette (page 238)
◆ Spinach Stuffed Shells (page 264)
◆ Steamed yellow squash
◆ Healthy Choice Bordeaux Cherry Chocolate Chip low-fat ice cream

◆ Low-fat vegetable soup
◆ Crustless Quiche (page 253)
◆ Greek Pilaf (page 272)
◆ Hard rolls
◆ Fat-free cookies

◆ Aspen Black Bean Soup (page 226)
◆ Steamed mixed vegetables

◆ Roasted new potatoes
◆ Fresh fruit

◆ Summer Vegetable Salad (page 236) with Very Green
   Dressing (page 237)
◆ Tofu Loaf (page 267)
◆ Wild rice
◆ Fat-free frozen yogurt topped with warmed lite apple pie
   filling

◆ Romaine, Boston lettuce and curly endive salad
◆ Vegetarian Chili (page 231) with baked tortilla chips
◆ Chile 'n Cheese Cornbread (page 221)
◆ Fresh raspberries topped with fat-free vanilla yogurt

◆ Minute Minestrone (page 229)
◆ Pasta with marinara sauce
◆ Steamed broccoli
◆ Fresh fruit

◆ Spinach salad with boiled egg white, mushrooms and
   toasted walnuts
◆ Spaghetti with Lentil Spaghetti Sauce (page 241)
◆ Stuffed "Med" Bread (page 223)
◆ Raspberry sorbet

◆ Minute Minestrone Soup (page 229)
◆ Vegetable Lasagna (page 268)
◆ Easy Peach Cobbler (page 278)

◆ Vegetable Salad (page 236) with Very Green Dressing
   (page 237)
◆ Millet Burgers with Mushrooms (page 258)
◆ Healthy Choice low-fat mint chocolate chip ice cream

◆ Mushroom and Barley Soup (page 230)
◆ Tofu Loaf with tricolored grilled peppers (page 267)
◆ Fresh fruit salad

◆ Tossed salad
◆ Vegetarian Pizza
◆ Chocolate Almond Dream (page 277)

◆ Coleslaw with Marzetti's Fat-Free Slaw Dressing
◆ Vegetarian Chili (page 231)
◆ Entenmann's fat-free pound cake with strawberries

◆ Black Bean, Corn and Barley Salad (page 232)
◆ Cheese Enchiladas (page 249)
◆ Fat-free hot fudge sundae

◆ Raw vegetables with fat-free Ranch dressing
◆ Stuffed Eggplant Creole (page 266)
◆ Bananas Foster (page 275)

◆ Oven Fried Zucchini Sticks (page 220)
◆ Pasta with Quick Alfredo Sauce (page 262)
◆ Tiramisu (page 279)

◆ Mexican Artichoke Dip with pita crisps (page 219)
◆ Bean and Rice Burritos (page 245)
◆ Fresh fruit salad with yogurt

◆ Baked potato
◆ Steamed mixed vegetables
◆ Lima beans with fat-free sour cream
◆ Fresh berry mix

◆ Tossed salad
◆ Bean and Cornbread Bake (page 244)
◆ Watermelon

◆ Sliced tomatoes with fresh basil and vinaigrette
◆ Spring Vegetables in Cream Sauce wrapped in tortillas (page 265)
◆ Waldorf salad made with fat-free mayonnaise

◆ Broccoli & cauliflower salad
◆ Rigatoni with Lentil Spaghetti Sauce (page 241)
◆ Fresh orange

◆ Grated Carrots in Vinaigrette (page 238)
◆ Mock Egg Foo Young
◆ Brown rice
◆ Easy Peach Cobbler (page 278)

About the Healthy Heart Formula Recipes

The recipes included here will get you started with healthy eating. However, there are many other great low-fat and vegetarian cookbooks—they are listed on page 292. We have provided some familiar recipes, like lasagna, that have been modified. In addition, we've included some items that may be new to you. All, though, are practical, so you won't find any recipes that take all day to cook. Many recipes call for canned and convenience items to cut your time in the kitchen.

Most of these recipes call for nonstick cooking spray like Pam. To cut the sodium in recipes, use no-salt-added tomato products. Rinsing other canned products will also cut the sodium.

Where a range of an ingredient is indicated, the lesser was used to analyze the recipe (as in 1 to 2 tsp. salt). Fiber content is listed when 3 grams or more. Enjoy!

Boursin Cheese Spread

This recipe is from More Low-fat Favorites *by Ceacy Thatcher. Try it with pita bread crisps, crackers, raw vegetables, or in crepes with veggies.*

Yield: 12 1/4-cup servings

8 oz. fat-free margarine
16 oz. fat-free cream cheese
2 cloves fresh garlic, minced, or 1 tsp. chopped garlic in jar
1/2 tsp. leaf oregano, dried
1/4 tsp. leaf marjoram, dried
1/4 tsp. leaf thyme, dried
1/4 tsp. leaf basil, dried
1/4 tsp. dill weed, dried
1/4 tsp. white pepper

1. Using a hand mixer or spoon, mix all ingredients until well blended.

2. Chill one hour before serving.

Nutrient Analysis per Serving:
40 calories
0.7 gram fat
5 grams protein
2.6 grams carbohydrate
373 mg. sodium

Cajun Garbanzo Nuts

This is a great substitute for nuts and they're good on a salad as well.

Yield: 4 1/3-cup servings

15 1/2 oz. can garbanzo beans
1 tsp. Cajun spice mix or spice mix you prefer

1. Preheat oven to 325°. Spray baking sheet with cooking spray.

2. Drain and rinse beans.

3. Spread beans close together on baking sheet.

4. Sprinkle 1/2 of spice mix over beans. Lay hands on top of beans and gently roll. Sprinkle remaining spice on.

5. Bake 45 to 55 minutes, testing often at the end of baking time to find the texture you prefer. Baking longer will produce a texture similar to corn nuts. Baking shorter will produce softer texture in the middle, chewy on the outside.

Nutrient Analysis per Serving:
83 calories
1.5 grams fat
4 grams protein
14 grams carbohydrate
4 grams fiber
338 mg. sodium

Mexican Artichoke Dip

*When company calls, this is a quick recipe
to throw together!*

Yield: 10 1/4-cup servings

2/3 cup fat-free mayonnaise
1/3 cup Parmesan cheese, freshly grated
1/4 tsp. hot pepper sauce
1/2 tsp. garlic powder
1 cup soft bread crumbs
2 14-oz. cans artichoke hearts, drained and chopped
4-oz. can green chiles, your choice of hotness! (for really
   mild tastebuds, use 1/2 can)

1. Preheat oven to 350°. Combine first 5 ingredients. Gently
fold in artichokes and green chiles.

2. Spray a 1-quart casserole dish with cooking spray. Spoon
dip mixture into dish and bake 20 minutes. Or microwave on
medium for 12 to 14 minutes.

3. Serve with baked pita bread triangles, fat-free tortilla
chips, or crackers.

Nutritional Analysis per Serving:
59 calories
1.1 grams fat
3 grams protein
9 grams carbohydrate
334 mg. sodium

Oven Fried Zucchini Sticks
Yield: 48 sticks, 4 servings

1/2 cup Italian bread crumbs
2 Tbsp. fat-free Parmesan cheese
1/4 tsp. garlic powder
3 medium zucchini
Water
1 cup fat-free or low-fat spaghetti sauce

1. Preheat oven to 475°. Spray cookie sheet with cooking spray.

2. Place bread crumbs, cheese, and garlic powder in a zip-lock bag; shake well to combine. Set aside.

3. Cut each zucchini lengthwise into 8 pieces; cut each piece in half lengthwise. Fill a saucer with water. Dip each zucchini stick in water and drop into bag of crumb mixture. Shake until coated on all sides, and place on cookie sheet. Repeat with rest of sticks.

4. Bake for 10 to 15 minutes or until brown and tender. Serve with warm spaghetti sauce.

Nutrient Analysis per Serving:
94 calories
1.2 grams fat
5 grams protein
17 grams carbohydrate
437 mg. sodium

Chile 'n Cheese Cornbread

Yield: 6 pieces

1 package Gold Medal Golden Cornbread & Muffin Mix
1/3 cup skim milk
2 egg whites
2 Tbsp. water
2 Tbsp. dry butter buds
1 Tbsp. (or more if you like) drained green chiles
1 clove or 1/2 tsp. chopped garlic
1/2 cup drained whole kernel corn
1/2 cup fat-free grated cheddar cheese

1. Preheat oven to 425°. Blend all except last 2 ingredients in bowl until just mixed. Gently stir in corn and cheese.

2. Pour into 8-inch round or square pan that has been sprayed with cooking spray. Sprinkle grated cheese on top. Bake 10 to 14 minutes.

Nutrient Analysis per Serving:

135 calories
1.3 grams fat
4 grams protein
28 grams carbohydrate
296 mg. sodium

Pumpkin Muffins

Yield: 12 muffins

2 egg whites
1 Tbsp. tub margarine
3/4 cup + 2 Tbsp. canned unsweetened pumpkin
2/3 cup brown sugar
3/4 cup skim milk
2 cups all-purpose flour
2 tsp. baking powder
1/2 tsp. baking soda
1/2 tsp. salt
1/4 tsp. ground ginger
1/2 tsp. each ground cinnamon and nutmeg
1/2 cup raisins (optional)

1. Preheat oven to 400°. In large bowl, combine egg whites, margarine, pumpkin, sugar, and milk. In small bowl combine remaining ingredients. Fold wet and dry ingredients together until just blended. Fold in optional raisins.

2. Spray loaf pan with cooking spray. Pour batter into pan and bake for 20 to 25 minutes. Remove from pan and cool on wire rack.

Serving suggestion:
Serve with Orange Cream Cheese Spread: Mix fat-free cream cheese, orange marmalade, and powdered sugar to taste.

Nutritional Analysis per Serving:
169 calories
4 grams protein
1.3 grams fat
214 mg. sodium

Stuffed "Med" Bread

This bread is a wonderful accompaniment with soup, salad, or Mediterranean dishes.

Yield: 5 2 1/2-inch slices

1/4 cup each water and red wine
8 sun dried tomato pieces
1/2 medium sized eggplant
1 clove garlic, minced
1/4 tsp. salt
1/2 tsp. basil
1/4 tsp. oregano
1 package Pillsbury Crusty French Loaf (found with canned biscuits)
1/4 cup tomato sauce

1. Preheat oven to 350°. Spray cookie sheet with cooking spray.

2. Boil water and wine together. Remove from heat and add tomatoes. Let sit several minutes until soft and hydrated.

3. Peel eggplant. Slice into 1/2-inch slices; cut each slice into 6 to 8 pieces.

4. Spray nonstick sauté pan with cooking spray. Add garlic and cook 1 to 2 minutes. Add eggplant, salt. and herbs and cook 5 minutes. Drain tomatoes. Add tomato sauce; stir and cover. Cook 5 to 10 minutes until eggplant is tender.

5. Open french loaf can and unroll loaf. Spoon eggplant mixture onto dough and spread out to within 1 inch of edge of dough. Roll up like a jelly roll and tuck each end of bread under. Place on cookie sheet.

continued on next page

Stuffed "Med" Bread (continued)

6. Bake for 30 to 35 minutes. Cool on wire rack 5 minutes before slicing.

Nutrient Analysis per Serving:
170 calories
6.7 grams protein
1.2 grams fat
33 grams carbohydrate
448 mg. sodium

Zucchini Bread

You won't believe it's fat free! Make two and freeze one!

Yield: 1 loaf, 12 slices

1 1/2 cups flour
1 tsp. cinnamon
1/2 tsp. ground nutmeg
1/2 tsp. baking soda
1/2 tsp. baking powder
1/4 tsp. salt
1 package of Butter Buds
2 egg whites
1/4 cup applesauce
3/4 cup sugar
1/4 tsp. dried grated orange rind
1/2 cup skim milk
1/2 tsp. vanilla
1 cup zucchini, unpeeled and grated
1/2 cup grape nuts (optional)

1. Preheat oven to 350°. Spray loaf pan with cooking spray.

2. Sift flour, cinnamon, nutmeg, soda, baking powder and salt. Add butter buds to mixture; set aside.

3. Mix egg whites, applesauce, sugar, orange rind, milk, and vanilla.

4. Add sifted ingredients and blend in grated zucchini. Add grape nuts if desired.

5. Pour into loaf pan and bake 60 to 70 minutes.

Nutrient Analysis per Serving:
113 calories
0.2 gram fat
2.6 grams protein
26 grams carbohydrate
108 mg. sodium

226   Aspen Black Bean Soup

A hearty, delicious soup that is great after a morning walk.

Yield: 6 1 1/3-cup servings

1 medium onion, chopped
3 cloves garlic, minced, or 3 tsp. chopped garlic in jar
1 tsp. dried whole oregano
1/2 tsp. dried whole thyme
1/2 tsp. cumin
1/4 tsp. cayenne pepper
2 15-oz. cans (3 cups) black beans, drained and rinsed
3 cups fat-free chicken broth
2 tomatoes, chopped
1/2 cup onion, chopped finely
1/2 cup fat-free grated mozzarella or cheddar cheese
  (optional)

1. Spray skillet with cooking spray. Cook onion and garlic until tender, about 5 minutes; add a little water if needed. Stir in spices; cook 2 to 3 minutes.

2. Place half the beans in blender and purée until smooth, adding broth as needed to help make smooth.

3. Add puréed beans and remaining broth and beans to onion mixture. Bring to boil and then lower to medium heat and simmer 20 to 30 minutes.

4. Serve garnished with diced tomatoes, onions, and cheese.

Serving suggestion:

For a complete meal, add a salad, and cornbread or a grilled vegetable sandwich.

Nutritional Analysis per Serving:

144 calories	1.3 grams fat
8.4 grams protein	26 grams carbohydrate
449 mg. sodium	8 grams fiber

Leek and Potato Soup

Yield: 16 servings

8 potatoes
4 medium carrots
2 lbs. of leeks
2 cups evaporated skim milk
Salt & pepper to taste

1. Peel potatoes and carrots. Cut leeks down the center and rinse thoroughly. Cut all vegetables into 1-inch pieces.

2. Place all vegetables into large pot of hot water. Bring to a boil and simmer, covered, for 45 minutes, or until potatoes and carrots are tender. Since carrots take longer, you may start them off first in the pot.

3. Drain 90 percent of the water off. Purée in batches in blender with small amounts of milk in each batch.

4. Place all puréed soup back in the pot. Stir well, adding additional milk if needed.

Nutrient Analysis per Serving:
141 calories
0.3 gram fat
6 grams protein
30 grams carbohydrate
75 mg. sodium (with no salt added)

Lentil Soup

Yield: 6 1 1/2-cup servings

2 medium onions, chopped
6 large crushed garlic cloves
2 stalks celery, chopped
7 cups water
1 cup fat-free chicken broth
1 pound dry lentils
1/2 tsp. basil
1 1/2 tsp. thyme and oregano
1 bay leaf
1 to 2 tsp. salt
Lots of freshly ground black pepper
2 to 3 medium carrots, sliced
Red wine vinegar, and chopped tomatoes to garnish on top

1. Brown onions, garlic, and celery in a pan sprayed with cooking spray, adding 1 Tbsp. of water as needed.

2. Place water, lentils, herbs, and salt in a kettle. Bring to a boil, lower heat to a very slow simmer, and cook, covered, for 20 to 30 minutes.

3. Add black pepper and carrots. Cover, and let simmer another 30 to 45 minutes, stirring occasionally.

4. Remove bay leaf. Serve hot, with a sprinkle of red wine vinegar and chopped tomatoes on top of each bowlful.

Nutritional Analysis per Serving:
182 calories
0.7 gram fat
13 grams protein
33 grams carbohydrate
612 mg. sodium
9 grams fiber

Minute Minestrone Soup

Yield: 4 1 1/2-cup servings

5 oz. frozen spinach, thawed
1 medium carrot, diced
8-oz. can tomato sauce
1 cup water
1/2 tsp. onion powder
14 1/2-oz. can diced tomatoes
1/2 tsp. garlic powder
1 cup green beans
1 tsp. Italian seasoning
1 cup cooked pasta
1/2 tsp. dried basil
14-oz. can kidney beans, drained
1 tsp. dried or 2 Tbsp. fresh minced parsley

1. Combine all ingredients in a 1 1/2-quart saucepan.

2. Simmer 10 to 15 minutes or until carrots are tender. Add more water for a thinner soup.

Variation

Omit green beans and carrots and add a 10 oz. package frozen mixed vegetables, adding more water if necessary.

Nutrient Analysis per Serving:

189 calories
2.1 grams fat
9 grams protein
38 grams carbohydrate
980 mg. sodium
8 grams fiber

Mushroom and Barley Soup
Yield: 6 1 1/2-cup servings

1/2 cup uncooked pearl barley
4 1/2 cups water
1 medium onion, chopped
2 medium cloves garlic, minced
1 lb. mushrooms, sliced
3 cups fat-free chicken broth
3 to 4 Tbsp. dry sherry
Freshly ground black pepper

1. Place the barley and 1 1/2 cups of the water in a large saucepan. Bring to a boil, cover, and simmer until the barley is tender (20 to 30 minutes).

2. Meanwhile, heat 1 to 2 Tbsp. of water in a skillet. Add the onions and sauté for about 5 minutes over medium heat; add garlic and mushrooms. Cover and cook, stirring occasionally, until everything is very tender, about 10 to 12 minutes.

3. Add the sauté with all its liquid to the cooked barley, along with the remaining 2 cups of water and chicken broth. Grind in a generous amount of black pepper, and simmer, partially covered, another 20 minutes over very low heat. Add sherry, season to taste, and serve.

Nutritional Analysis per Serving:
97 calories
0.4 gram fat
3.3 grams protein
18 grams carbohydrate
348 mg. sodium
3 grams fiber

Vegetarian Chili

Yield: 6 1 1/2-cup servings

1 medium onion, chopped
2 large cloves garlic, minced
1 medium zucchini or 1 medium bell pepper, chopped
28-oz. can crushed tomatoes in purée
15-oz. can tomato sauce
15-oz. cans kidney beans, drained
2 to 4 tsp. chili powder
2 tsp. cumin
1/2 tsp. oregano
1/4 cup uncooked bulgur wheat
Finely minced parsley, tomato, and onion for topping
Cayenne pepper or black pepper to taste

1. Heat a small amount of water in a nonstick pot. Add onion and garlic. Sauté over medium heat about 5 to 10 minutes. Add zucchini or bell pepper, and sauté until all the vegetables are tender.

2. Add the tomatoes, tomato sauce, beans, spices, and bulgur. Simmer over lowest heat, stirring occasionally, for 15 minutes. Taste to adjust seasonings. Serve hot, topped with parsley, chopped fresh tomato, and onion if desired.

Serving suggestions:
- ◆ Over baked tortilla chips with fat-free cheddar cheese stirred in
- ◆ Rolled up in a flour tortilla
- ◆ Stuffed in a bell pepper

Nutritional Analysis per Serving:

220 calories	12 grams protein
1056 mg. sodium	1.0 gram fat
44 grams carbohydrate	11 grams fiber

Black Bean and Corn Salad

Yield: 4 1-cup servings

1 cup corn, drained
16-oz. can black beans, drained and rinsed
1/2 cup fat-free Italian dressing
1/2 cup plain nonfat yogurt
1/2 tsp. cumin
1/8 tsp. garlic powder
Pepper to taste
2 cups romaine lettuce, torn
2 tomatoes, quartered
2 Tbsp. fat-free cheddar cheese (optional)

1. Mix corn, beans, and dressing. Marinate in refrigerator at least 30 minutes. Mix yogurt and spices. Add pepper to taste. Set aside.

2. Spoon bean mixture over lettuce. Top with yogurt sauce or serve on the side. Garnish with tomato quarters and tortilla chips. Sprinkle with cheese if desired.

Variation

Add 1/2 cup cooked barley and 1 to 2 Tbsp. additional dressing to corn and black bean mixture.

Serving suggestion

Serve with baked tortilla chips or make your own by cutting corn tortillas into quarters, spray with cooking spray, and sprinkle with spices. Bake at 375° until crispy, turning once.

Nutritional Analysis per Serving

155 calories	7.8 grams protein
289 mg. sodium	0.8 gram fat
30 grams carbohydrate	8 grams fiber

Fiesta Pasta Salad

*This is Shirley Lippincott's recipe for a great quick meal
and a good way to use leftover pasta and vegetables.
Besides the pasta and vegetables, you can be creative!
Throw in whatever you have in the refrigerator or pantry.*

Yield: 4 2 1/2-cup servings

1 pound bag of frozen "fiesta style" vegetables
4 cups cooked pasta (rotini or wheels work nicely)
14-oz. can artichoke hearts, drained, quartered
1 large tomato, cut in chunks
15-oz. can beans, your choice
1 1/2 cups fat-free salad dressing

1. Thaw vegetables for several hours or run warm water over
to thaw.

2. Mix and all ingredients gently until blended.

3. For best taste, refrigerate for at least 30 minutes to let
flavors blend.

Nutritional Analysis per Serving:
344 calories
1.6 grams fat
13 grams protein
67 grams carbohydrate
312 mg. sodium
10 grams fiber

Jicama and Orange Salad
Yield: 4 3/4-cup servings

2 navel oranges, peeled, sectioned, and cut in two; or 1 can
   mandarin orange segments, drained and rinsed
2 cups jicama, julienne-cut
3 Tbsp. orange juice
2 Tbsp. rice vinegar
Leaf lettuce

1. Combine oranges and jicama in a bowl.

2. Mix together juice and vinegar. Toss lightly with orange
mixture.

3. Chill before serving. Serve over lettuce leaf.

Nutritional Analysis per Serving:
93 calories
2 grams protein
0.1 gram fat
3 mg. sodium
2.5 grams fiber

Oriental Salad

Yield: 4 1 1/2-cup servings

4 cups shredded romaine lettuce
1 celery stalk, finely chopped
1 to 2 green onions, sliced
1/2 cup sliced water chestnuts, rinsed
10-oz. package frozen snow peas, thawed or steamed and
    cooled
1 teaspoon sesame seeds
1/2 cup mung bean sprouts
11-oz. can mandarin oranges (optional)

Dressing
3/4 cup white wine vinegar
1/4 cup sugar
1/2 tsp. sesame oil
1 tsp. soy sauce
1/4 tsp. pepper

1. Toss salad ingredients. Mix together dressing and toss with salad.

Nutrient Analysis per Serving:
85 calories
1.1 grams fat
2 grams protein
19 grams carbohydrate
102 mg. sodium

Summer Vegetable Salad

Pick a mixture of vegetables from below to suit your taste.
Use about 1 to 1 1/2 cups total vegetables per person.
Beets
Bell peppers (all colors)
Broccoli
Cabbage (green and red)
Carrots
Cauliflower
Celery
Cucumber
Fresh herbs
Green beans
Radishes
Red onion
Scallions
Snow peas
Spinach
Sprouts
Yellow squash
Zucchini
Tomatoes and mushroom slices as toppings

1. Peel when necessary; mince or grate everything and mix
well. Serve with Very Green Dressing (next page).

Very Green Dressing

Yield: 4 1/3-cup servings

1 Tbsp. chopped, packed parsley
5 medium-large fresh spinach leaves
1 cup 1% or fat-free buttermilk
1 medium clove garlic
1/2 tsp. salt
1 tsp. lemon juice
1/4 cup fat-free sour cream
12 medium fresh basil leaves
1/2 of a small zucchini, cut in chunks

1. Purée all ingredients in a blender or food processor and mix with salad.

Nutritional Analysis per Serving—summer vegetable salad and dressing:
80 calories
5 grams protein
375 mg. sodium
0.9 gram fat
14 grams carbohydrate
3 grams fiber

Vegetables in Vinaigrette

It is a French tradition to have grated vegetables in vinaigrette as a starting course.

Yield: 4 servings

Use the following amounts of one or more vegetables:
7 finely grated carrots
1/2 finely grated celery root (now available in the U.S., also called celeriac)
2 thinly sliced cucumbers
1/3 head finely grated red cabbage

Add:
1/2 cup fat-free vinaigrette (strong flavored best)
1/4 cup finely chopped parsley
Salt and pepper to taste

1. Combine all ingredients. Let marinate at least 30 minutes.

2. For a variation, add 1 to 2 Tbsp. fat-free sour cream to vinaigrette.

Nutritional Analysis per Serving:
30 calories
0.1 gram fat
0.5 gram protein
7.3 grams carbohydrate
51 mg. sodium

Curry Sauce

Yield: 6 1/4-cup servings

10 oz. silken low-fat tofu
1 to 2 cloves garlic, minced
1/4 cup skim milk
1/2 tsp. cumin
1 to 2 tsp. curry powder
1 Tbsp. ketchup
1/2 tsp. salt
1/4 tsp. garam masala
Pepper to taste

1. Blend all in blender. Heat over stovetop or in microwave until warmed through.

Note

Garam masala is a spice blend found in gourmet shops and large health food stores. If not found, you can replace with 2 pinches of cinnamon, 1 pinch of ground cardamom, and 1 pinch of ground cloves.

Serving suggestions

◆ Serve over rice or vegetables, or as topping on crepes.
◆ Try with a mixture of: cauliflower, peas, and potatoes; spinach or eggplant; potatoes, peas, or green beans; or lentils and tomatoes.

Nutritional Analysis per Serving:
21 calories
0.6 gram fat
3.5 grams protein
0.8 gram carbohydrate
225 mg. sodium

240 Dijon Sauce

Yield: 4 1/4-cup servings

1/2 cup fat-free sour cream
1/2 cup plain nonfat yogurt
1 to 2 Tbsp. Dijon style mustard
Salt, pepper, and garlic powder to taste

1. Mix all ingredients. Heat until just warm—do not boil.

Serving suggestions
Great over vegetables, for a dipping sauce for fresh
artichokes, over crepes, or with roasted or baked potatoes.

Nutritional Analysis per Serving:
43 calories
0.1 gram fat
2.5 grams protein
66 mg. sodium

Lentil Spaghetti Sauce

Yield: 8-1 cup servings

1 medium onion, chopped
1 green pepper, chopped
5 cloves garlic, minced
3 cups fat-free beef broth
1 1/2 cups water
1-lb. bag dry lentils
1/2 to 1 tsp. crushed red pepper flakes
2 3/4 tsp. Italian seasoning
1/2 tsp. onion powder
1/2 tsp. salt
1 Tbsp. vinegar
28-oz. can no-added-salt stewed tomatoes
2 15-oz. cans low-sodium tomato sauce
Freshly ground pepper to taste

1. Spray a Dutch oven with cooking spray. Add, onion, pepper, and garlic. Sauté over medium heat until tender, adding 1 to 2 Tbsp. of water as necessary.

2. Add broth, water, lentils, red pepper, Italian seasoning, onion powder, and salt. Bring to a boil. Cover, reduce heat and simmer 45 to 60 minutes, until lentils are tender.

3. Stir in vinegar, tomatoes, and tomato sauce. Bring to a boil, reduce heat, and simmer 30 minutes or until desired consistency is obtained. Stir often.

Leftover idea

Purée some leftover sauce in blender and you have Lentil Sloppy Joes! You may need to add additional tomato sauce to taste.

continued on next page

Lentil Spaghetti Sauce (continued)

Nutritional Analysis per Serving:
270 calories
0.9 gram fat
18 grams protein
49 grams carbohydrate
826 mg. sodium
7 grams fiber

Roasted Red Pepper Sauce

Yield: 5 1/3-cup servings

1/2 green onion, chopped
1/4 tsp. garlic powder
1 heaping cup roasted red peppers (can be bought in a jar)
2 Tbsp. white wine vinegar (can be flavored)
1/3 cup fresh parsley, torn into pieces
1/3 cup nonfat yogurt or fat-free sour cream

1. Purée all ingredients except yogurt in food processor. Place in microwave-safe dish and cook on medium-high for 2 minutes.

2. Fold in yogurt or sour cream. Heat another 30 seconds on high. Serve with vegetables, or over vegetable crepes, veggie burgers or grilled tofu.

Nutritional Analysis per Serving:
25 calories
0.1 gram fat
1 gram protein
5 grams carbohydrate
16 mg. sodium

244 Bean and Cornbread Bake
Yield: 4 servings

1/3 cup each: chopped green pepper, celery, and onion
3 cups cooked or canned beans (pinto, black beans, kidney
    beans, or any combination)
8 oz. tomato sauce
2 Tbsp. ketchup
1 tsp. dry mustard
1/4 tsp. pepper
1 package Gold Medal corn muffin mix
2 Tbsp. honey
2 egg whites
1/3 cup skim milk
1/4 cup grated fat-free cheddar cheese (optional)

1. Preheat oven to 375°. Spray pan with cooking spray. Add pepper, celery, and onion with 1 to 2 Tbsp. water and cook until tender. Add beans, tomato sauce, ketchup, dry mustard, and pepper.

2. Mix muffin mix with honey, egg whites, and milk. Stir until just blended. Fold in cheese, if desired.

3. Spray 2-quart baking dish with cooking spray. Put bean mixture in dish, and top with cornbread batter. Bake 30 to 35 minutes until bread is golden brown.

Nutritional Analysis per Serving:
471 calories
2.7 grams fat
21 grams protein
95 grams carbohydrate
814 mg. sodium
7 grams fiber

Bean and Rice Burritos

Yield: 6 servings

12 small reduced-fat flour tortillas
2 16-oz. cans flavored refried beans, such as Rosarita's Zesty
    Salsa Fat-Free Refried Beans
3 cups cooked brown rice
Cumin, chili powder, and cayenne pepper to taste
1 head romaine lettuce, shredded
3 to 4 scallions, chopped
2 ripe tomatoes, chopped
Fat-free or oil-free Mexican salsa

1. Preheat oven to 350°. Wrap tortillas, 6 each, in aluminum foil, sprinkling with a few drops of water before wrapping up. Bake 10 to 15 minutes. (Tortillas can also be warmed in microwave for 2 to 3 minutes but become tougher.)

2. Put beans and cooked rice in a saucepan. Add spices to taste. Heat 5 to 10 minutes. Meanwhile, prepare the vegetables.

3. Place bean mixture down the middle of each tortilla. Top with lettuce, scallions, tomato, and salsa. Tuck in the top and bottom edges, roll into a burrito, and serve immediately, topped with additional salsa to taste.

Nutritional Analysis per Serving:
440 calories
4.6 grams fat
15 grams protein
87 grams carbohydrate
11 grams fiber

Black Bean Enchilada Casserole

*This quick and easy casserole was modified from
Janet Boyd's recipe.*

Yield: 4 servings

15-oz. can Southwestern style black beans (with spices),
    undrained
15-oz. can Del Monte chili-style tomatoes
1/4 cup picante sauce
3 corn tortillas
4-6 oz. fat-free cheddar cheese

1. Preheat oven to 350°. In bowl, mix beans, tomatoes, and sauce. Spray 2-quart round casserole dish with cooking spray.

2. Place 1 corn tortilla in bottom of dish. Add 1/3 of bean mixture, 1/3 of cheese, another tortilla, 1/3 of bean mixture, another tortilla and rest of bean mixture.

3. Bake 20 minutes. Sprinkle remaining 2 Tbsp. cheese on during last 5 minutes of cooking.

4. To enlarge this recipe for a 9 x 13 pan, use 3 cans of black beans, 3 cans of tomatoes, and 12 tortillas, overlapping 6 tortillas on each layer.

Low-sodium variation:
Cook 1 sliced onion, 1 tsp. chopped garlic, and 1 sliced bell pepper until tender. Add 15 oz. can stewed tomatoes and 3/4 cup picante sauce. Use 1 1/2 cups cooked black beans with 1 1/2 tsp. cumin and 1 tsp. chili powder.

Nutritional Analysis per Serving:
250 calories
1.7 grams fat
1211 mg. sodium
20 grams protein
39 grams carbohydrate
10 grams fiber

Boston Baked Beans

Yield: 6 1 1/4-cup servings

1 medium onion, chopped
2 medium sized, tart apples, peeled and
    cut into small chunks
16-oz. can tomatoes, chopped
2 Tbsp. maple syrup
1 Tbsp. vinegar
1 Tbsp. soy sauce
1 Tbsp. parsley flakes
1 1/2 tsp. dry mustard
1 1/4 tsp. powdered ginger
1/2 tsp. ground cinnamon
1/4 tsp. black pepper
3 to 4 Tbsp. molasses
5 cups cooked white beans or pinto beans

1. Sauté the onion in a small amount of water until soft. Add the remaining ingredients, except for the beans. Cook and stir for about 5 minutes.

2. Preheat oven to 350°. Stir beans into mixture, and transfer to a deep casserole or a 9 x 13 baking pan. Cover tightly with foil, and bake for 30 to 45 minutes.

3. Serve warm with rice, cornbread, or warmed tortillas.

Nutritional Analysis per Serving:
272 calories
1.2 grams fat
13 grams protein
322 mg. sodium
10 grams fiber

Broccoli and Tofu Stir-Fry

Yield: 4 1 1/2-cup servings

2 Tbsp. chicken broth
2 tsp. grated fresh ginger
3 cloves garlic, minced
3 green onions, chopped
3 cups chopped fresh broccoli
1 Tbsp. vinegar
1 Tbsp. hoisin sauce
2 Tbsp. reduced sodium soy sauce
1/4 cup water
1 lb. firm tofu, crumbled into smaller than bite size pieces

1. Heat chicken broth in a nonstick pan. Add ginger, garlic, and green onions. Sauté 2 minutes. Add broccoli, and stir-fry until broccoli is tender crisp. Add more chicken broth or water to pan if necessary.

2. Mix together vinegar, hoisin sauce, soy sauce, and water. Set aside. Add tofu to broccoli, and stir-fry 2 more minutes. Add sauce mixture and continue cooking until warmed through.

3. Serve over brown rice, bulgur, or noodles.

Nutritional Analysis per Serving:
117 calories
2.5 grams fat
15 grams protein
11 grams carbohydrate
383 mg. sodium
3 grams fiber

Cheese Enchiladas

This recipe is from More Low-fat Favorites
by Ceacy Thatcher.

Yield: 12 enchiladas

1/2 medium onion, chopped
1 clove garlic, minced
1/2 tsp. ground cumin
1/2 tsp. chili powder
Pinch of salt
2 cups fat-free chicken broth
15-oz. can no-added-salt tomato sauce
12 small corn tortillas
12 oz. fat-free grated cheddar cheese
1/2 cup fat-free sour cream or yogurt cheese

1. Spray skillet with cooking spray. Sauté onions and garlic until tender and brown. Stir in spices; then add chicken broth and tomato sauce. Stir and bring to a boil. Reduce heat and simmer for 15 minutes until thickened.

2. Preheat oven to 375°. Spray a 9 x 13 pan with cooking spray. Fill each corn tortilla with about 1/4 cup cheese and two teaspoons sour cream. Roll up and place seam side down. Spray enchiladas with cooking spray, and bake 5 to 7 minutes. Ladle enchilada sauce over the enchiladas, and return to the oven for 5 to 7 more minutes.

3. Serve with shredded lettuce and Spanish rice.

Nutritional Analysis per Serving:
275 calories
27 grams protein
826 mg. sodium
2.4 grams fat
37 grams carbohydrate
4 grams fiber

250   Colorado Stuffed Peppers

Yield: 4 servings

3 roma tomatoes, or 2 medium tomatoes, chopped coarsely
2 green onions, chopped
1/4 medium red onion, chopped
1 to 2 cloves garlic, minced
1/2 sweet red pepper, chopped
1 cup cooked brown rice or bulgur
2 cups cooked black beans or canned black beans
1 tsp. cumin
1/4 cup fat-free cheddar cheese
4 bell peppers, seeded and cored

1. Spray pan with cooking spray. Sauté tomatoes, onions, garlic, and red pepper in 1 Tbsp. water until cooked to desired tenderness.

2. Add brown rice or bulgur, black beans, cumin, and cheese to pan, and gently stir until warm and cheese is melted.

3. Meanwhile, cover whole peppers and cook in microwave until tender crisp, about 5 minutes (cook longer for softer peppers). Fill peppers with bean mixture. Garnish with chopped red pepper, if desired.

Nutritional Analysis per Serving:
217 calories
1 gram fat
16 grams protein
39 grams carbohydrate
121 mg. sodium
7 grams fiber

Crepes

*Impress your guests with this versatile French meal that
is as easy to make as pancakes!*

Yield: 20 crepes

2 cups white flour
2 egg whites
2 Tbsp. sugar
1/4 tsp. salt
2 cups skim milk, divided
1 tsp. vanilla (omit for main dish or vegetable-filled crepes)
1 cup + 2 Tbsp. water

1. Place flour, egg whites, sugar, salt, 1 cup milk, and vanilla
in bowl. Mix well by hand or with beater. While still mixing,
add in 1 cup milk and water. Beat at medium speed until
well mixed.

2. Spray a 10-inch nonstick skillet with cooking spray. Place
skillet on stovetop over medium-high heat. When pan is hot,
pour a scant 1/4 cup of batter into pan, turning pan at the
same time to cover. (It's all in the wrist!)

3. Cook 1 1/2 minutes until bottom of crepe is golden brown.
Use plastic spatula to gently lift up sides of crepe. You can
then either turn the crepe with the spatula or flip the crepe
up in the air and over. Cook 30 more seconds until other side
is brown.

Note:

It is important to use a pan that is unscratched to keep
crepes from sticking. The first crepe is never perfect and
usually goes to the dog! After making a batch of crepes, you
will learn which thickness and cooking time you prefer. The
batter can be saved for up to a week in the refrigerator. The

continued on next page

Crepes (continued)

batter will separate, so when ready to use again, mix with wire whip or electric beater. Cooked crepes can be kept in the refrigerator or freezer by layering between wax paper.

Fillings:

BREAKFAST/DESSERT:
◆ Fleishman's liquid nonfat margarine or Ultra Fat-Free Promise
◆ Honey, jam, granulated or powdered sugar, cinnamon sugar
◆ Fresh or canned fruit of your choice (sliced strawberries, bananas, and blueberries work well)
◆ Canned pie filling
◆ Liqueur such as triple sec, amaretto, or kahlua
◆ Fat-free yogurt or sorbet

LUNCH/BRUNCH/DINNER:
◆ Spring Vegetables in Cream Sauce (page 265)
◆ Delightful Spinach (page 271)
◆ Ratatouille (page 274)
◆ Steamed Vegetables with Curry Sauce (page 239)
◆ Vegetables and prepared low-fat spaghetti sauce
◆ Flavored black beans and salsa
◆ Filling from Spinach Stuffed Shells (page 264)
◆ Tofu filling from Vegetable Lasagna (page 268)
◆ Vegetables of your choice

Nutritional Analysis per Serving (4 crepes, no filling):
244 calories
0.7 gram fat
10 grams protein
48 grams carbohydrate
180 mg. sodium

Crustless Quiche

Yield: 4 servings

10 egg whites
1 cup evaporated skim milk
1 tsp. Italian seasoning
1/3 tsp. salt
1/4 tsp. garlic powder
10-oz. package spinach, thawed
4 oz. fat-free mozzarella cheese, shredded

1. Preheat oven to 350°.

2. Beat egg whites, milk, and spices together until frothy. Fold in spinach and cheese.

3. Spray 10-inch pie pan with cooking spray. Pour egg mixture into pan and bake for 45 to 50 minutes.

Variation:
Use 1 cup of any leftover vegetables. Add water chestnuts and low sodium soy sauce for oriental flavor.

Nutritional Analysis per Serving:
170 calories
0.3 gram fat
26 grams protein
15 grams carbohydrate
750 mg. sodium

Faux Fajitas

Yield: 3 servings

2 Tbsp. water
1 medium onion, cut in half, then sliced
1 to 2 cloves fresh garlic, minced
1/2 tsp. chili powder
1 tsp. cumin
1/4 tsp. pepper
1 medium red pepper, sliced thinly
8-oz. package Seitan, traditionally seasoned (found in
   refrigerated section of natural foods store)
6 small flour tortillas
Lettuce, tomato, onion, salsa, fat-free cheese,
   fat-free sour cream

1. Preheat oven to 350°. Heat 2 Tbsp. water over medium heat. Add onion and garlic; cook 3 to 4 minutes. Add spices and red pepper and cook until vegetables are tender, adding more water if necessary. Add drained seitan and cook another 5 minutes.

2. Stack tortillas and sprinkle top one with a few drops of water. Wrap in foil and bake until warm—about 10 minutes.

3. To serve, fill a tortilla with seitan-veggie mixture. Top with shredded lettuce, chopped tomato, onion, salsa, cheese, and sour cream.

Nutritional Analysis per Serving:
322 calories
27 grams protein
163 mg. sodium
3.7 grams fat
45 grams carbohydrate
3 grams fiber

Happy Family Dinner

Yield: 8 1 1/2-cup servings

Vegetables:
1 lb. cubed firm tofu (optional)
1/2 cup fat-free chicken broth
4 cloves fresh garlic, minced
3 tsp. fresh ginger, minced
4 green onions, sliced
4 cups broccoli florets
1 1/2 cups sliced carrots
2 cups sliced mushrooms
2 cups thinly sliced bok choy
2 cups snow peas
1/2 cup sliced water chestnuts
1 cup whole baby corn, canned

Sauce:
1 1/2 cups fat-free chicken broth
2 to 3 Tbsp. dry sherry
1 to 2 Tbsp. soy sauce
3 Tbsp. cornstarch
Small amount white pepper

1. Combine sauce ingredients in a separate bowl and set aside.

2. Brown optional tofu in nonstick pan for 5 to 10 minutes.

3. Place broth in a wok or large saucepan. Heat until it boils; add garlic, ginger, and green onions. Cook 2 minutes. Then add broccoli, and carrots. Cook and stir for about 10 minutes. Add mushrooms, bok choy, and snow peas. Cook and stir for 3 to 5 minutes. Add water chestnuts and cook a few more minutes.

continued on next page

Happy Family Dinner (continued)

4. Add sauce mixture to pan. Bring to a boil, stirring constantly. After mixture boils and thickens, stir in baby corn; add optional tofu.

Serving suggestion:

Serve over brown rice or noodles.

Nutritional Analysis per Serving:
117 calories
6.2 grams protein
578 mg. sodium
0.9 gram fat
24 grams carbohydrate
5.7 grams fiber

Hoppin' John

Yield: 4 1 3/4-cup servings

1 medium onion, chopped
1 bay leaf
1 tsp. dried thyme
1/2 tsp. pepper
1 to 2 Tbsp. water
10-oz. package frozen sliced okra, thawed (optional)
16-oz. can kidney beans
16-oz. can black-eyed peas
3 cups cooked bulgur or brown rice

1. Spray pan with cooking spray. Add onion and spices. Add 1 to 2 Tbsp. of water and cook until onion is tender. (If using okra, add here and cook 5 minutes until warm.) Add beans and peas with their liquid. Simmer 10 minutes or more.

2. Stir in bulgur. Cook until warmed through.

Nutritional Analysis per Serving:

326 calories
1.5 grams fat
17 grams protein
65 grams carbohydrate
718 mg. sodium
11 grams fiber

Millet Burgers

Patty Magliato introduced us to millet with this recipe.
It's even a favorite with kids!

Yield: 8 small burgers; 4 servings

1 cup millet, uncooked
1/8 tsp. cayenne pepper, or other spice
2 cups water
1 tsp. salt (optional)
1 cup grated carrot
1/2 cup onion, minced
1/2 cup fresh parsley, minced
1/2 to 3/4 cup whole wheat flour

1. Spray skillet with cooking spray. Heat over medium heat briefly; add millet and spice. Roast until fragrant, 2 to 3 minutes.

2. Add water and salt; bring to a boil. Simmer until water is absorbed, 35 to 40 minutes.

3. Preheat oven to 375°. Pour millet into a bowl and let cool. Add last 4 ingredients and mix with a spoon or hands. Form into 8 patties.

4. Bake 10 minutes on each side.

5. Serve on a bun with all the trimmings.

Nutritional Analysis per Serving:
219 calories
7 grams protein
17 mg. sodium
1.8 grams fat
45 grams carbohydrate
9 grams fiber

Mock Egg Foo Yung

Yield: 8 2-oz. patties

16 oz. low-fat firm tofu, crumbled
2 egg whites
6 Tbsp. cornmeal or seasoned bread crumbs
1 Tbsp. low-salt soy sauce
3/4 tsp. fresh ginger, finely grated
4 green onions, finely chopped
2 large cloves garlic, finely minced
1/4 tsp. sesame oil
1 medium sized carrot, finely grated
1/2 cup mung bean sprouts, cut in half
1 Tbsp. sesame seeds

1. Squeeze out extra water from tofu. Mix all ingredients except last 3. Fold in last ingredients until just blended. Form into 8 small patties.

2. Spray pan with cooking spray. Cook patties on both sides until lightly browned.

3. Serve with sweet and sour sauce, teriyaki sauce, or sauce from Happy Family Dinner (page 255).

Nutritional Analysis per Serving:
135 calories
3.3 grams fat
12 grams protein
15 grams carbohydrate
269 mg. sodium

Oat Nut Burgers
Yield: 6 burgers

2/3 cup rolled oats (not instant)
1/3 cup chopped cashews
1 onion, chopped
3 stalks celery, chopped
2 carrots, grated (or 1 carrot and 1/3 zucchini, grated)
1/4 cup each whole wheat flour and water
1 tsp. low-sodium soy sauce (optional)
Salt and pepper to taste

1. Mix all ingredients. Season to taste with soy sauce or salt and pepper.

2. Shape into 6 burgers. Cook in pan sprayed with cooking spray—about 10 minutes on each side, or broil in oven.

3. Serve on a bun with all the trimmings.

Nutritional Analysis per Serving:
117 calories
4.4 grams fat
4 grams protein
15 grams carbohydrate
24 mg. sodium
3 grams fiber

Pasta e Fagiol
Yield: 6 servings

32 oz. prepared low-fat pasta sauce
8-oz. can "pasta ready" Italian-style tomatoes
2 15-oz. cans water-packed red kidney beans, drained and
  rinsed
1 tsp. Italian seasoning
1 to 2 cloves garlic, minced
1 pound uncooked egg-free whole wheat or spinach pasta

1. Preheat oven to 350°. Place all the ingredients except the
pasta in a large bowl. Stir until blended. Cook the pasta sepa-
rately according to directions, and drain.

2. Combine the sauce with the pasta in a 3-quart casserole
dish and bake for 20 minutes.

Nutritional Analysis per Serving:
437 calories
3.3 grams fat
20 grams protein
86 grams carbohydrate
13 grams fiber

Pasta With Quick Alfredo Sauce

Yield: 4 2-cup servings

1 1/2 cups fat-free cottage cheese
1/2 cup skim milk
1/2 tsp. garlic powder or 2 cloves fresh garlic, pressed
1 package butter buds
2 Tbsp. freshly grated parmesan cheese
2 dashes nutmeg
10-oz. package frozen peas, thawed
6 cups cooked pasta

1. Purée all ingredients except peas and pasta in food processor or blender.

2. Pour into microwave-safe dish and cook on medium-high for 2 minutes. Or cook on stove, over medium-low heat, until warm.

3. Toss pasta with peas. Pour sauce over pasta.

Nutritional Analysis per Serving:
421 calories
2.6 grams fat
26 grams protein
72 grams carbohydrate
443 mg. sodium
5 grams fiber

Sloppy Joes

Yield: 4 servings

1 cup TVP (Textured Vegetable Protein) (found in bulk at
  large natural food stores)
1 cup boiling water
16-oz. can sloppy joe sauce
4 whole wheat hamburger buns

1. To rehydrate the TVP, place the TVP in a medium
saucepan and pour boiling water over it.

2. Add the sloppy joe sauce to the TVP; cook over low heat
until heated thoroughly.

3. To serve, pour the TVP mixture over the hamburger rolls.

Nutritional Analysis per Serving:
198 calories
2 grams fat
15 grams protein
32 grams carbohydrate
804 mg. sodium

Recipe from The Simple Soybean And Your Health *by Mark
Messina and Virginia Messina. © 1994. Published by Avery
Publishing Group, Inc., Garden City Park, New York.
Reprinted with permission.*

Spinach Stuffed Shells

Yield: 4 servings

1/2 lb. large pasta shells, cooked until slightly firm
10-oz. package frozen spinach, cooked and drained
1 cup fat-free cottage cheese
1/2 cup grated fat-free mozzarella cheese
2 Tbsp. freshly grated Parmesan cheese
2 cloves garlic, minced
1 1/2 tsp. Italian seasoning
1/2 tsp. pepper
2 cups low-fat spaghetti sauce

1. Mix spinach, cheeses, and spices until well blended.

2. Stuff each shell with spinach mixture, and top with sauce.

3. Bake at 350° for 10 to 15 minutes or microwave until hot.

Nutritional Analysis per Serving:
360 calories
3 grams fat
28 grams protein
55 grams carbohydrate
967 mg. sodium
4 grams fiber

Spring Vegetables In Cream Sauce

Yield: 4 1-cup servings

Sauce:

1 1/2 cups fat-free chicken broth
1 cup skim milk
3 Tbsp. cornstarch
1 package butter buds
1/2 tsp. tarragon
1/4 tsp. each dill and basil
1/2 tsp. onion powder
1/2 tsp. garlic salt
1 tsp. lemon pepper
1 tsp. lemon juice

Vegetables:

1-lb. package Green Giant California-style vegetables (cauli-
    flower, carrots, asparagus) or other vegetable mixture
7- or 14-oz. can artichoke hearts, quartered
1/2 red bell pepper, sliced thinly

1. Put chicken broth, milk, cornstarch, and butter buds in
blender. Blend on high until mixed well. Pour into large
saucepan. Add rest of sauce ingredients. Cook over medium
heat, stirring often until thick.

2. Meanwhile, steam vegetables or cook in microwave. Add
to thickened sauce.

Serving Suggestions:

Serve over rice, bulgur, or angel hair pasta. Or roll up in a
crepe or flour tortilla.

Nutritional Analysis per Serving:

103 calories	0.4 gram fat
5.5 grams protein	22 grams carbohydrate
550 mg. sodium	4 grams fiber

266 Stuffed Eggplant Creole

Yield: 4 servings

2 small eggplants (1 lb. each)
1 clove garlic, crushed
1/4 cup each: finely chopped onion, green pepper, celery
1 lb. firm tofu, cubed
14-oz. can tomatoes, undrained
1/4 tsp. salt
1/4 tsp. thyme
Tabasco or cayenne (optional)
1 cup dry bread crumbs, plain or Italian
1 cup fat-free sour cream or nonfat yogurt

1. Preheat oven to 375°. Wash eggplant, cut in half lengthwise. Place in a large pan, and cover with water. Bring to a boil and cover. Simmer 15 minutes. Drain and cool.

2. Scoop out pulp from eggplant, taking care to leave 1/4 inch of the shell intact. Set aside.

3. Spray a nonstick skillet with cooking spray. Add vegetables and cook until tender crisp. Add tofu and cook until warm.

4. Stir in tomatoes, salt, thyme, and Tabasco if desired. Add half of the bread crumbs. Stir in eggplant and sour cream.

5. Stuff mixture back into the 4 eggplant shells. Top with remaining bread crumbs. Place in baking dish and bake for 30 minutes.

Nutritional Analysis per Serving:
290 calories
3.5 grams fat
49 grams carbohydrate
5 grams fiber

Tofu Loaf

*This recipe is from Norma Robinson. The pecans give it
an interesting texture and flavor.*

Yield: 8 slices

16 oz. low-fat firm tofu
1/4 cup chopped pecans
1/2 cup canned tomatoes, chopped
2 egg whites
1/4 cup skim milk
1/2 cup dry bread crumbs, plain or seasoned
1/2 tsp. salt
1/2 tsp. each onion and garlic powder
1 tsp. thyme, cumin, oregano, or Italian seasoning
Optional seasonings: chopped parsley, green onion, finely
   chopped celery or onion.

1. Preheat oven to 350°. Squeeze out excess liquid from tofu,
and crumble. With a spoon, mix with rest of ingredients until
well blended. Pour into loaf pan that has been sprayed with
cooking spray. Bake 50 to 60 minutes.

2. Serve like meat loaf with ketchup, salsa, or pasta sauce or
on a bun like a burger. Leftovers are great as sandwiches.

Nutritional Analysis per Serving:
86 calories
8 grams protein
5 grams carbohydrate
4.2 grams fat
346 mg. sodium

Vegetable Lasagna

This recipe was inspired by Patty Magliato. It uses uncooked noodles to save time.

Yield: 9 servings

Marinara Sauce:

2 28-oz. cans Progresso Italian-style tomatoes with basil
28-oz. can no-added-salt tomato sauce
3 to 4 large cloves garlic, minced
2 tsp. basil
2 tsp. Italian seasoning
Pinch sugar
Salt and pepper to taste

Lasagna:

2 pounds firm low-fat tofu
1/4 cup lemon juice
1 Tbsp. honey
2 to 3 cloves garlic, minced
1 tsp. fennel seeds
1 tsp. each dried oregano and basil
10-oz. package frozen broccoli, thawed
1 medium zucchini, sliced thinly
2 carrots, grated
8-oz. package regular or whole wheat lasagna noodles

1. To make sauce, pour both cans of tomatoes in food processor or blender. Process until smooth. Pour into saucepan and add remaining sauce ingredients. Simmer 15 to 20 minutes.

2. While sauce is cooking, squeeze extra liquid from tofu. Put in food processor; add lemon juice, honey, garlic, and spices. Process until well mixed. In microwave safe dish, gently mix vegetables together. Cover and cook in microwave 6 to 8 minutes, until tender. Pour into colander to drain excess liquid.

continued on next page

3. Preheat oven to 375°. To assemble, spray 9 x 13 inch pan with cooking spray. Do not cook noodles. Spread 1 cup of the sauce in the bottom of the pan. Lay down 3 noodles side-by-side. Spread 1 cup of sauce. Spread 1/2 of tofu and 1/2 of vegetable mixture. Add 1 cup of sauce. Add 3 noodles and press down. Spread 1 cup of sauce over noodles, then spoon the remaining tofu and vegetables. Top with 1 cup of sauce. Lay down last of noodles and press down. Cover with remaining sauce, making sure that all noodles are covered.

Nutritional Analysis per Serving:
236 calories
2.2 grams fat
15 grams protein
41 grams carbohydrate
413 mg. sodium
5 grams fiber

Bulgur and Veggie Mix
Yield: 5 1-cup servings

2 cups water
1/4 tsp. salt
2 1/2 cups chopped broccoli, or other vegetable in season
1 cup dry bulgur
1/2 tsp. thyme

1. Bring water to boil. Add salt and thyme. Add broccoli. Simmer 5 minutes.

2. Place bulgur in heat-proof serving bowl. Pour water and broccoli over bulgur.

3. Cover and let sit until most of the water is absorbed.

4. Pour off excess water and fluff with a fork.

Variation:
Any vegetable or combination of vegetables, fresh or frozen, can be used in place of the broccoli. California-style vegetable mix (frozen) also works well.

Nutritional Analysis per Serving:
103 calories
0.5 gram fat
5.6 grams protein
22 grams carbohydrate
148 mg. sodium
6 grams fiber

Delightful Spinach

Yield: 4 1-cup servings

8 oz. fat-free cream cheese
1 tsp. mixed herbs (Italian seasoning, herbs de Provence, etc.)
2 10-oz. packages frozen chopped spinach, thawed or cooked, or 2 lb. fresh spinach or other green, cooked
Pepper, to taste
2 drops Tabasco sauce (optional)

1. In a nonstick saucepan, cook cream cheese and spices together until melted. Squeeze out excess water from spinach. Add to cream cheese.

2. Cook until warmed through.

Serving Suggestion:
Serve over rice, on pizza, or stuffed in a crepe or tortilla.

Nutritional Analysis per Serving:
76 calories
0.2 gram fat
11 grams protein
9 grams carbohydrate
466 mg. sodium

Greek Pilaf

Yield: 7 2/3-cup servings

1 1/2 cups long-grain brown rice
2 1/2 cups water
1 1/2 cups minced onion
1 small stalk celery, minced
1/2 tsp. salt
1/2 cup sunflower seeds or pine nuts
1 tsp. black pepper
4 medium cloves garlic, minced
2 Tbsp. lemon juice
1/4 cup freshly minced parsley
1 Tbsp. dried mint

1. Place the rice and water in a saucepan. Bring to a boil, cover, and simmer until tender (40 to 45 minutes).

2. Heat 2 Tbsp. of water in a small skillet. Add onion, celery, and salt, and sauté until tender, adding more water as necessary (5 to 8 minutes). Add sunflower seeds or pine nuts, black pepper, and garlic. Sauté for 5 minutes.

3. Stir the sautéed mixture into the cooked rice along with the lemon juice and herbs. Mix well.

Time Saver:
Use bulgur wheat instead of rice, and cook 10 minutes. Or use instant brown rice.

Nutritional Analysis per Serving:
194 calories
3.7 grams fat
5 grams protein
36 grams carbohydrate
162 mg. sodium
3 grams fiber

Oven Fried Potatoes

Yield: 4-6 servings

6 medium potatoes, (peeled or unpeeled), sliced thinly
Your choice of seasonings: garlic powder, Italian seasoning,
   cajun spice mix, chili powder and cumin, seasoned salt,
   Mrs. Dash

1. Preheat oven to 350°. Spray cookie sheet with cooking spray.

2. Place potatoes on cookie sheet, spray lightly with cooking spray, and sprinkle with desired spices. Bake for about 20 minutes or to desired brownness, turning once.

3. For extra-crisp potatoes, slice paper thin. For "home fries" slice thicker or in wedges.

Nutritional Analysis per Serving:
217 calories
0.2 gram fat
4.6 grams protein
50 grams carbohydrate
11 mg. sodium
5 grams fiber

Ratatouille

Yield: 8 1-cup servings

1 eggplant, peeled and cut into 1-inch cubes
4 cloves garlic, crushed
8 tomatoes, quartered
3 zucchini, sliced
1 cup sliced mushrooms
1 tsp. oregano
1 tsp. basil
Salt and pepper to taste

1. Spray nonstick pan with cooking spray. Brown eggplant, adding 1 tablespoon of water at a time as needed. Cook until tender. Add remaining ingredients.

2. Cook over medium heat until vegetables are tender, stirring frequently.

3. Reduce heat, cover, and simmer 10 to 15 minutes. Remove cover and continue cooking until most of the liquid has evaporated.

Nutrient Analysis per Serving:
58 calories
1 gram fat
2 grams protein
12 grams carbohydrate
15 mg. sodium
4 grams fiber

Bananas Foster

Yield: 6 servings

1 package butter buds
2 Tbsp. orange juice
1 Tbsp. lemon juice
3 Tbsp. water
2/3 cup brown sugar
4 bananas, cut in half lengthwise
3 to 4 Tbsp. dark rum
1 tsp. cinnamon

1. Mix butter buds, orange juice, lemon juice, and water in nonstick skillet. Add brown sugar, and cook until thick and bubbly, stirring often. Add bananas, spooning sauce over until warm. Add rum. Let warm a few seconds. Tilt the pan slightly and touch lighted match to inside edge of pan. The liquor will be ignited for a few seconds. For a more dramatic effect, sprinkle cinnamon over flame to create "sparks."

2. Serve over nonfat vanilla frozen yogurt.

Nutritional Analysis per Serving (bananas and sauce only):
191 calories
0.4 gram fat
1 gram protein
45 grams carbohydrate
9 mg. sodium

Caramel Dip

This is Cindy McKee's recipe for a dip you won't believe is fat-free! Try with sliced apples or other fresh fruit or on graham crackers.

Yield: 8 2-Tbsp. servings

8 oz. fat-free cream cheese
1/3 cup brown sugar, packed
1 tsp. Watkin's caramel flavor
1 tsp. vanilla

1. Mix all ingredients with mixer. Chill and serve.

Nutrient Analysis per Serving:
57 calories
0 fat
4 g. protein
11 grams carbohydrate
192 mg. sodium

Note: Watkins caramel flavor can be ordered by calling 1-800-247-5907, Director #47233.

Chocolate Almond Dream

Yield: 5 3/4-cup servings

8 oz. fat free cream cheese
1/2 to 1 cup powdered sugar (start with 1/2 cup and increase
   to taste)
3/4 tsp. almond extract
1/2 cup Cool Whip Lite
1 3/4 cups skim milk
1 small package instant chocolate pudding mix
1/4 cup crushed graham crackers, grapenuts or fat-free
   granola

1. In small bowl, beat cream cheese until smooth. Add powdered sugar and almond extract and mix well. Fold in Cool Whip.

2. In another small bowl, mix milk and pudding mix according to package directions.

3. In wine or dessert glasses, put small amount of pudding, a larger layer of cream cheese mixture and another layer of chocolate pudding. Top with graham cracker crumbs or other crunchy topping.

4. Refrigerate at least 1/2 hour before serving.

Nutritional Analysis per Serving:
275 calories
3.2 grams fat
9 grams protein
54 grams carbohydrate
722 mg. sodium

Easy Peach Cobbler

Yield: 6 servings

1 cup flour
2/3 cup sugar
1 1/2 tsp. baking powder
1/2 tsp. salt
1 package butter buds (not diluted)
1 tsp. almond flavoring
3/4 cup canned evaporated skim milk
21-oz. can lite peach pie filling

1. Preheat oven to 350°. Spray 2-quart casserole dish with cooking spray.

2. Mix together flour, sugar, baking powder, salt, butter buds, almond flavoring, and milk. Pour into casserole.

3. Spoon pie filling on top.

4. Bake at 350° for 35 to 40 minutes or until golden brown.

Serving Suggestion:
Serve warm with nonfat frozen yogurt.

Variation:
Blueberry or apple pie filling also work well. If you like a lot more fruit than crust, use 2 cans of pie filling and put into dish first, topped with batter.

Nutritional Analysis per Serving:
275 calories
4.6 grams protein
0.4 gram fat
64 grams carbohydrate

Tiramisu

This light dessert is great for company.

Yield: 8 servings

8 oz. fat-free cream cheese
1/2 cup fat-free sour cream
2/3 cup powdered sugar
1/3 cup sugar
3 Tbsp. water
2 egg whites
3/4 cup hot water
1 1/2 Tbsp. sugar
1 Tbsp. + 1 tsp. instant coffee granules
1/4 cup kahlua or other coffee liqueur
15 ladyfingers
3 Tbsp. unsweetened cocoa

1. Mix cream cheese, sour cream, and powdered sugar in a bowl at high speed with electric mixer.

2. In the top of a double boiler over simmering water, combine next 3 ingredients. Beat at high speed until stiff peaks form. Gently fold in 1/4 of egg white mixture into cream mixture. Gradually fold in rest of egg white mixture.

3. Combine next 4 ingredients in small bowl. Arrange 15 ladyfinger halves, cut side up in 8 x 8 pan (size of ladyfingers may vary, so you may need more or less to cover pan). Drizzle 1/2 of coffee mixture over ladyfinger halves. Spread half of cream cheese mixture over ladyfingers. Repeat procedure with remaining ladyfingers and cream cheese mixture.

4. Sprinkle cocoa over top, using sifter or strainer. Place one toothpick in each corner and cover with plastic wrap. Chill or freeze 2 hours before serving.

continued on next page

Tiramisu (continued)

Nutritional Analysis per Serving:
196 calories
0.8 gram fat
7 grams protein
37 grams carbohydrate
317 mg. sodium

Very Berry Shake

Yield: 2 1-cup servings

1 cup frozen sweetened berries, any combination
   (blueberry and strawberry is good)
1 cup nonfat vanilla yogurt

1. Blend all and serve.

Variation:

You can also use any combination of any fruit, fresh or frozen. If using fresh, freeze first. Cut the sugar by using sugar-free yogurt and unsweetened berries. Good combinations of fruit include:

◆ Banana and strawberry
◆ Pineapple and coconut flavoring
◆ Apple and apple pie spice
◆ Chocolate syrup and frozen nonfat yogurt

Nutritional Analysis per Serving:
189 calories
0.2 gram fat
6 grams protein
44 grams carbohydrate
71 mg. sodium

CHAPTER FIFTEEN

CHOICES

Your life is filled with choices. Some of them got you where you are today. Others may lead you to reverse heart disease, and the disease of the spirit that lingers inside. Your future will be affected by the choices you make today.

Learn to make choices that are best for your overall happiness and well-being. Learn from your mistakes. Keep the big picture in mind.

Many people are miserable today because of bad choices: in business, in love, in health. The natural order is so resilient, however, that they often get a second chance. As my friend Paul Smith always says, "Opportunity only knocks three or four times!"

Our bodies are built for survival. As human beings we can and should expect more than survival. Good health and happiness can be achieved. You don't have to be caught, trapped in the hamster's cage. If your life has no meaning, there is no incentive to make life-enhancing choices. As our society has become more segmented, you may lose the drive to strive. Open up to new ideas. Enjoy life to the fullest!

At the Preventive Health Institute, we have helped people like you make some of the healthy choices. We encourage you to make life-enhancing choices. Others have found good health and happiness. So can you!

Making Good Choices

◆ *Will I be happy, or will I settle for content?*

◆ *Is my glass half-full or half-empty? Do I have an upbeat attitude?*

◆ *Will I be fit or fat?*

◆ *Will the practice of self-awareness and control govern my actions, or will stress make me explode?*

◆ *Will I live as a human being, with all the blemishes, or will I always expect perfection?*

◆ *Should I eat to live, or continue to live to eat?*

◆ *Should I use my body, and improve in health, or lose it, and get even sicker?*

◆ *Am I happy with myself, with who I really am? If not, what am I willing to change?*

◆ *Should I continue to put up with abuse from my spouse and family?*

◆ *Should I cut back and enjoy life, or continue to "kill myself" for my work or my boss?*

◆ *Does my life have meaning?*

Stress reduction and group support help people like you work
through and resolve these dilemmas. Practice making the right
choices for you!

Take this test:

At the end of your natural life, after the funeral, at the grave,
what will you want on your tombstone?

♦ "I didn't work hard enough."
♦ "I didn't gather enough toys."
♦ "I didn't get to eat everything I wanted."

or

♦ "I loved my spouse, my family, my community."
♦ "I died having experienced great happiness."
♦ "I contributed all I possibly could during my short life, and
 I hope others will say it was enough."

When a loved one develops a terminal illness, they feel a
heightened sense of being. They develop the ability to live life to
the fullest, savoring all that comes in their path. No event seems
too small or insignificant to enjoy!

Your time is short. Why not focus on what is important, and
with all your energy, work toward that personal goal. Don't be
diverted, just do it!

After you determine what is important, I hope this book helps
make you "feel like doing it." There are many ways to live life.
Since we only go around once, why not feel good about it? Only
you can answer that question. What is the meaning of life for you?

Postscript

We are most interested in what you choose and how you come to "feel like doing it." After you read this book, please write us with your comments, and share your success with others. Then fill out and return this survey:

1. Have you found your motivation to change?

2. Where did you find it?

3. How have you changed your eating habits, exercise routine, outlook on life?

4. How have the changes you instituted made life different?

5. Are you healthy and happy?

Frank Barry, MD
c/o Preventive Health Institute
2130 Hollowbrook
Colorado Springs, Colorado 80918
or fax: (719) 590-7037

REFERENCES

1. Ornstein R, Sobel D. *Healthy Pleasures.* New York: Addison-Wesley; 1989.
2. Ornish DM. "The Lifestyle Heart Trial." *Lancet.* 1990; 336:129-133.
3. Watts GF, et al. "Effects on coronary artery disease... in the St. Thomas atherosclerosis regression study." *Lancet.* 1992; 339:563-569.
4. Gould, Ornish, et al. "Changes in myocardial perfusion abnormalities by positron emission tomography after long-term, intense risk factor modification." *JAMA.* 1995; 274: 894-961.
5. The Coronary Drug Project Research Group. "Clofibrate and niacin in coronary heart disease..." *JAMA.* 1975; 231:360-381.
6. The pravastatin multinational study group for cardiac risk patients. "Effects of pravastatin..." *Am J Cardiol.* 1993; 72(14):1031-1037.
7. Brown G. "Regression of coronary artery disease..." *N Engl J Med.* 1990; 323(19):1289-1298.
8. Blankenhorn DH, et al. "Beneficial effects of combined colestipol-niacin therapy..." *JAMA.* 1987; 257:3233-3240.
9. Pedersen T. Scandinavian simvastatin study group. "The Scandinavian simastatin survival study." *Lancet.* 1994; 344:(45)1383-1389.
10. Shepherd J, et al. "Prevention of coronary heart disease with pravastatin in men with hypercholesterolemia." *N Engl J Med* 1995; 333: 1301-1307.
11. Kannel WB, Abbott RD. "Incidence and prognosis of unrecognized myocardial infarction: an update on the Framingham study." *N Engl J Med.* 1984; 311(18):1144.

288

12. Hamm CW. "A randomized study of coronary angioplasty compared with bypass surgery..." *N Engl J Med.* 1994; 331:(16)1037-1043.

13. Kimmel, SE, et al. "The relationship between coronary angioplasty procedure volume and major complications." *JAMA.* 1995; 274:1137-1142.

14. Ridolphi RL. "The relationship between coronary artery lesions and myocardial infarcts: ulceration of atherosclerotic plaques precipitating coronary thrombosis." *Am Heart J.* 1977; 93(4):468-486.

15. Arca M, et al. "Hypercholesterolemia in postmenopausal women." *JAMA.* 1994; 271(6):453-59.

16. SHEP Cooperative Research Group. "Prevention of stroke by antihypertensive drug treatment..." *JAMA.* 1991; 265(24):3255-64.

17. Unpublished study, American Heart Association Meeting, University of Washington at the AHA, 1995.

18. Depres JP, et al. "Hyperinsulinemia as an independent risk factor for ischemic heart disease." *N Engl J Med* 1996; 334:952-957.

19. *Cardiovascular Horizons,* 1996; 5:11+.

20. Hunninghake DB, et al. "The efficacy of intensive dietary therapy." *N Engl J Med.* 1993; 328(17):1213-19.

21. Giovanucci E, et al. "A prospective study of dietary fat and risk of prostate cancer." *J Natl Cancer Inst.* 1993; 85(19):1571-9.

22. Howe GR, et al. "Dietary factors and risk of breast cancer." *J Natl Cancer Inst.* 1990; 82(7):561-69.

23. Gould KL, et al. "Short term cholesterol lowering." *Circulation.* 1994; 89(4):1530-38.

24. Fischer L. "The Low Cholesterol Gourmet" quoted in the *Colorado Springs Gazette Telegraph.* Sept. 28, 1994; p: 2 Lifestyle section.

25. Zemel MB. "Calcium utilization: effect of varying level and source of dietary protein." *Am J Clin Nutr.* 1988; 48:880-883.

26. Campbell W, et al. "Increased protein requirements in elderly people." *Am J Clin Nutr.* 1994; 60:50-9.

27. Stephens, NG, et al. "Randomized control trial of vitamin E..." *Lancet,* 1996; 347:781-786.

28. Zemel MB. "Calcium utilization: effect of varying level and source of dietary protein." *Am J Clin Nutr.* 1988; 48:880-883.

29. Kerstetter JE, Allen LH. "Dietary protein increases urinary calcium." *J Nutr.* 1990; 120:134-136.

30. Frahm A. *A Cancer Battle Plan.* Colorado Springs, CO; Pinon Press; 1992.

31. Verrillo A, et al. "Soybean protein diets in the management of Type II hyperlipoproteinemia." *Atherosclerosis*. 1985; 54:321-331.
32. Bresslau NA. "Relationship of animal protein-rich diet to kidney stone formation and calcium metabolism." *J Clin Endocrinol Metab*. 1988; 66:140-146.
33. Miettinen, TA, et al. "Reduction of serum cholesterol with sitostanolester margarine in a mildly hypercholesterolemic population." *N Engl J Med*, 1995; 333:1308-1312.
34. Havala S, Clifford M. *Simple, Lowfat and Vegetarian; Unbelievably Easy Ways to Reduce the Fat in Your Meals*. Baltimore; MD: Vegetarian Resource Group; 1994.
35. Green LA, Ruffin MT. "A closer examination of sex bias." *J Fam Pract*. 1994; 39:(4)331-6.
36. Douglas, PS, et al. "The evaluation of chest pain in women." *N Engl J Med*, 1996; 334:1311-1315.
37. Shaw LJ, et al. "Gender differences in the noninvasive evaluation of..." *Ann Int Med*. 1994; 120:(7)559-66.
38. Weaver, WD, et al. "Comparisons of characteristics and outcomes among women and men with acute myocardial infarction treated with thrombolytic therapy." *JAMA*, 1996; 275:777-782.
39. Stampfer MJ, et al. "A prospective study of postmenopausal estrogen therapy." *N Engl J Med*. 1985; 313;1044-9.
40. The PEPI Trial Group. "Effects of estrogen or estrogen-progestin regimens on heart disease risk factors in postmenopausal women." *JAMA*. V1995; 273:199-208, 1995.
41. Bush TL et al. "Cardiovascular mortality and noncontraceptive use of estrogen in women." *Circulation*. 1987; 75(6):1102-1109.
42. Walsh, BW, et al. "Effect of postmenopausal estrogen replacement on the concentrations and metabolism of plasma liproproteins." *N Engl J Med*. 1991; 325:1196-1204.
43. Grodstein, F, et al. "Postmenopausal estrogen and progestin use and the risk of cardiovascular disease." *N Engl J Med*, Vol. 1996; 335:453-461.
44. Riggs BL, Seeman E. "Effect of the fluoride-calcium regimen on vertebral fracture in postmenopausal osteoporosis." *N Engl J Med*. 1982; 306(8):446-450.
45. National Institute of Health Consensus Conference. "Optimal calcium intake." *JAMA*. 1994; 272(24):1942.
46. "Cancer Statistics." *CA Cancer Clinical Journal* 1994; 44: 7-26.
47. Gambrell, RD. *The Menopause*. London: Blackwell Scientific Publications Ltd.; 1988: 247.

48. Dupont WD, Page DL. "Menopausal estrogen replacement therapy and breast cancer." *Arch Intern Med.* 1991; 151:(1)67.

49. Stanford, JL, et al. "Combined estrogen and progestin hormone replacement therapy in relation to risk of breast cancer in middle aged women." *JAMA.* 1995; 274:137-142.

50. Colditz, GA, et al. "The use of estrogens and progestins and the risk of breast cancer in postmenopausal women." *N Engl J Med,* vol. 332, p. 1589, 1995; 332:1589-1593.

51. Jiang, W, et al. "Mental stress-induced myocardial ischemia and cardiac events." *JAMA.* 1996; 275:1651-1656.

52. Moliterno DJ, et al. "Coronary vasoconstriction." *N Engl J Med.* 1994; 330(7):454-9.

53. Kawachi I, et al. "Symptoms of anxiety and risk of coronary heart disease." *Circulation.* 1994; 90(5):2225-29.

54. Carney RM, et al. "Major depressive disorder predicts cardiac events in patients with coronary artery disease." *Psychosom Med.* 1988; 50(6):627.

55. Prochaska JO. "The transtheoretical model." *Am Psychol.* 1992; 47:1102-1114.

56. *Surgeon General's Report on Physical Exercise,* U.S. Government, 1996.

57. Kelly G. "Antihypertensive effects of aerobic exercise." *Am J Hypertens.* 1994; 7:115-119.

58. Blair SN, et al. "Physical fitness and all cause mortality." *JAMA.* 1989; 262(17):2395-2401.

59. Glynn TJ. *The Fagerstrom Tolerance Test in How to Help Your Patients Stop Smoking.* Washington D.C.: National Institute of Health; 1990. NIH publication 90-3064.

60. Selhub J, et al. "Vitamin status as primary determinants of homocysteinemia in an elderly population." *JAMA.* 1993; 270(22):2693-98.

61. Stampfer MJ, et al. "Vitamin E consumption and the risk of coronary artery disease in women." *N Engl J Med.* 1993; 328(20):1444-49.

62. Stephens, et al "Randomized controlled trial of vitamin E in patients with coronary disease: Cambridge Heart Antioxidant Study (CHAOS)."

63. Hodis, HN, et al. "Serial coronary angiographic evidence that antioxidant vitamin intake reduces progression of coronary artery atteroschlerosis. *JAMA,* 1995; 273:1849-1854.

64. Kushi, et al. "Dietary antioxidant vitamins and death from coronary heart disease in postmenopausal women." *N Eng J Med.* 1996: 334:1156-1162.

65. Selhub J, et al. "Association between plasma homocysteine concentrations and extracranial carotid artery stenosis." *N Engl J Med.* 1995; 332(5):286-291.

66. Morrison, HI, et al. "Serum folate and risk of fatal coronary heart disease." *JAMA*, 196; 275:1893-1896.

67. Press R, et al. "The role of chromium picolinate on serum cholesterol and apolipoprotein factions in human subjects." *West J Med.* 1990; 152:41-45.

68. Reiser S, et al. "Indices of copper status in humans." *Am J Clin Nutr.* 1985; 42(2):242-251.

69. Kessler D. "Therapeutic class wars—drug promotion in a competitive marketplace." *N Engl J Med.* 1994; 331(20):1350-1353.

70. Alavanja MC, et al. "Saturated fat intake and lung cancer risk." *J Natl Cancer Inst.* 1993; 85(23):1906-1916.

71. Chiu, et al. "Diet and risk of non-Hodgkin lymphoma in older women." *JAMA*. 1996; 275:1315-1321.

72. Howe GR, et al. "Dietary factors and risk of breast cancer." *J Natl Cancer Inst.* 1990; 82(7):561-69.

73. Giovannucci E, et al. "A prospective study of dietary fat and risk of prostate cancer." *J Natl Cancer Inst.* 1993; 85(19):1571-79.

74. Trock B, et al. "Dietary fiber, vegetables, and colon cancer." *J Natl Cancer Inst.* 1990; 82(8):650-61.

SUGGESTED READINGS

Foreword

The works of Nathan Pritikin.

The many books by Kenneth Cooper, MD.

The works of John McDougall, MD, and Mary McDougall.

Frahm A. *A Cancer Battle Plan.* Colorado Springs, CO: Pinon Press; 1992.

Ornish D. *Reversing Heart Disease.* New York. Ballantine; 1990.

Chapter 1—21st Century Medicine

Ornstein D, Sobel R. *Healthy Pleasures.* New York: Addison-Wesley, 1989.

Jones PH, Gotto AM Jr. "Prevention of Coronary Heart Disease in 1994." *Heart Dis Stroke.* 1994; 3(6):290-6.

Chapter 2—The Problem with Heart Disease

Kessler D. "Therapeutic class wars—drug promotion in a competitive marketplace." *N Engl J Med.* 1994; 331(20):1350-1353.

Arca M, et al. "Hypercholesterolemia in postmenopausal women." *JAMA.* 1994; 271(6):453-59.

Pekkanen J, et al. "Ten year mortality." *N Engl J Med.* 1990; 322(24):1700-1707.

Hunninghake DB, et al. "The efficacy of intensive dietary therapy..." *N Engl J Med.* 1993; 328(17):1213-19.

Bachinsky WB. "Angioplasty in Multivessel Coronary Artery Disease." *Hosp Pract Off Ed.* 1994; 29(12):27-33.

SHEP Cooperative Research Group. "Prevention of stroke by antihypertensive drug treatment." *JAMA.* 1991; 265(24):3255-64.

Ginsburg HJ. *From The Heart: Overcoming the Mental and Physical Trauma of Open Heart Surgery*. Denver: American Heart Association of Colorado; 1993.

Chapter 3—
The Practical Way to Reverse Blocked Arteries!

Hunninghake DB, et al. "The efficacy of intensive dietary therapy..." *N Engl J Med*. 1993; 328(17):1213-19.

Giovannucci E, et al. "A prospective study of dietary fat and risk of prostate cancer." *J Natl Cancer Inst*. 1993; 85(19):1571-79.

Gould KL, et al. "Short term cholesterol lowering." *Circulation*. 1994; 89(4):1530-38.

Morris DL et al. "Serum carotenoids and coronary heart disease." *JAMA*. 1994; 272(18):1439-1441.

White R and Frank E. "Health effects and prevalence of vegetarianism." *West J Med*. 1994; 160:465.

Chapter 4—Eating Right, the Practical Guide

Frahm A. *A Cancer Battle Plan*. Colorado Springs: Piñon Press; 1992.

Debakey M. *The Living Heart Brand Name Shoppers Guide*. New York: Mastermedia Limited; 1993.

Bellerson K. *The Complete and Up to Date Fat Book*. Garden City Park, NY: Avery Publishing Group; 1993.

Moran V. *Get the Fat Out: 501 Simple Ways to Cut the Fat Out of Any Diet*. New York: Crown; 1994.

Paino J, Messinger L. *The Tofu Book; The New American Cuisine*. Garden City Park, NY: Avery Publishing Group; 1991.

Havala S, Clifford M. *Simple, Lowfat and Vegetarian: Unbelievably Easy Ways to Reduce the Fat in Your Meals*. Baltimore: Vegetarian Resource Group; 1994.

Chapter 5—
The Fat Free Eater's Guide to the Grocery Store

The New Food Label, Food and Drug Administration, 1993.

Chapter 6—Eating Away from Home

Warshaw H. *The Healthy Eater's Guide to Family and Chain Restaurants*. Minnetonka, MN: Chronimed, 1993.

Day B. *Fast Facts on Fast Food for Fast People*. Louisville, KY: An Apple A Day Publishing. 1995.

Jacobson M, Fritschners. *The Fast Food Guide, Rev & Updated*. New York: Workman; 1991.

Chapter 7—
Women and Heart Disease—The Weaker Sex?

Gambrell RD. *The Menopause*. London: Blackwell Scientific Publications, Ltd; 1988; 247-261.

Green LA, Ruffin MT. "A closer examination of sex bias..." *J Fam Pract.* 1994; 39:(4)331-6.

Shaw LJ, et al. "Gender differences in the noninvasive evaluation of..." *Ann Int Med.* 1994; 120:(7)559-66.

Preuss HG. "Nutrition and diseases of women: cardiovascular disorders." *J Am Coll Nutr.* 1993; 12(4):417-425.

Peberdy MA, Ornato JP. "Coronary artery disease in women." *Heart Dis Stroke.* 1992; 1(5):315-19.

Nelson HD, et al. "Smoking, alcohol, and neuromuscular and physical function of older women." *JAMA.* 1994; 272(23):1825-31.

Eaker E, et al. "Cardiovascular disease in women." *Circulation.* 1993; 88: 1999.

Chapter 8—So What's Stopping You?

Moliterno DJ, et al. "Coronary vasoconstriction..." *N Engl J Med.* 1994; 330(7):454-9.

Kawachi I, et al. "Symptoms of anxiety and risk of coronary heart disease." *Circulation.* 1994; 90(5):2225-29.

Carney RM, et al. "Major depressive disorder predicts cardiac events in patients with coronary artery disease." *Psychosom Med.* 1988; 50(6):627.

Homes S. "The social readjustment rating scale." *J of Psychosom Res.* 1967; 11:213-218.

Eliot RS and Breo DL. *Is It Worth Dying For?* New York: Bantam Books, 1986.

Jiang T. *Mental Stress Testing.* Oxford, England. American Psychosomatic Society, Elsevier Science Ltd. Pergamon Imprint; 1994.

Chapter 9—Move Your Body

Blair SN, et al. "Physical fitness and all-cause mortality." *JAMA.* 1989; 262(17):2396-2401.

Ainsworth BE. "Compendium of physical activities: classification of energy costs of human activities." *Med Sci Sports Exerc.* 1993; 25(1)71-8.

Anderson B. *Stretching.* Bolinas, CA: Shelter Publications, 1980.

Franklin S. "Exercise and cardiac complications." *The Physician and Sports Medicine.* 1994; (22)2.

Kelly G. "Antihypertensive effects of aerobic exercise." *Am J Hypertens.* 1994; 7:115-119.

Chapter 10—Kick the Habit

National Cancer Institute. *How to help your patients stop smoking;* 1994.
Matzen. *Clinical Preventive Medicine.* Mosby: St. Louis, MO; 1993.
Entire issue, *The Journal of Family Practice,* June 1992, vol. 34, no 6.
Entire issue, *JAMA* 1991; 266(22).
Glynn TJ. *How to Help Your Patients Stop Smoking.* Washington DC: National Institute of Health; 1990. NIH publication 90-3064.

Chapter 11—Should I Be Taking a Supplement?

National Institute of Health Consensus Conference, "Optimal Calcium Intake." *JAMA.* 1994; 272(24)1942.
McDougall J. *The McDougall Plan.* Clinton, NJ: New Win Publishing Inc.; 1983.
Selhub J, et al. "Vitamin status and intake as primary determinants of homocysteinemia in an elderly population." *JAMA.* 1993; 270 (22):2693-98.
Stampfer MJ, et al. "Vitamin E consumption and the risk of coronary artery disease in women." *N Engl J Med.* 1993; 328(20):1444-49.
Schardt D. "Phytochemicals: plants against cancer." *The Nutrition Action Health Letter.* 1994; 21(3):1.
Morris DL, et al. "Serum carotenoids and coronary heart disease." *JAMA.* 1994; 272(18):1439-1441.
Vita chart, Inc. 3611 Henry Hudson Parkway, #1d, Bronx, NY.
Messina M, Messina V. *The Simple Soybean and Your Health.* Garden City Park, NY: Avery Publishing Group; 1994.
Ulene A, Ulene V. *The Vitamin Strategy.* Berkeley: Ulysses Press; 1994.
Somer E. *The Essential Guide to Vitamins and Minerals.* New York: Harper Collins; 1992.

Chapter 12—Pharmaceuticals

Kessler D. "Therapeutic class wars—drug promotion in a competitive marketplace." *N Engl Med.* 1994; 331(20):1350-1353.
The fifth report... high blood pressure. Washington, DC: National Institute of Health; 1993. NIH publication no. 93-1088.
Second report on... high blood cholesterol in adults. Washington, DC: National Institute of Health; 1993. NIH Publication no. 93-3095.

Chapter 13—A Word On Cancer Prevention

Giovanucci E, et al. "A Prospective Study of Dietary Fat and Risk of Prostate Cancer." *J Natl Cancer Inst.* 1993; 85(19):1571-9.

Howe GR, et al. "Dietary factors and risk of breast cancer..." *J Natl Cancer Inst.* 1990; 82(7):561-69.

Trock B, et al. "Dietary fiber, vegetables, and colon cancer..." *J Natl Cancer Inst.* 1990; 82(8):650-61.

Chapter 14—Delightful, Delicious, Delectable Recipes

McDougall M. *The McDougall Health Supporting Cookbook.* New Win Publications Inc.: Berkeley; 1986.

Hinman B, Snyder M. *Lean and Luscious and Meatless.* Rocklin, CA: Prima; 1992.

Gilliard J, Kirkpatrick J. *Beyond Alfalfa Sprouts and Cheese; The Healthy Meatless Cookbook.* Minnetonka, MN: Chronimed; 1993.

Baird P. *Quick and Hearty Meatless Microwave Meals Everyone Will Enjoy.* New York: Henry Holt; 1991.

Lakhani. *Indian Recipes for a Healthy Heart.* Los Angeles: Fahil Publishing; 1991 (this book is 75% vegetarian).

Woodruff S. *The Secrets of Fat Free Baking.* Garden City Park, NY: Avery Publishing Group; 1994.

Mateljan G. *Baking Without Fat.* Irwindale, CA: Health Valley Foods; 1994.

American Soybean Association, *free recipes and information about soy products.* 1-800-TALK-SOY.

Vegetarian Resource Group, nonprofit group devoted to vegetarianism; publishes magazine and books. (410)-366-VEGE

Chapter 15— Choices

Ornish DM. "Can lifestyle changes reverse coronary heart disease?" *Lancet.* 1990; (336):129.

INDEX

Acarbose, 23
ACE inhibitors, 22
additives, 191-192
aerobic exercise, 166
aging, 12, 27
alcohol, appetite and, 106
alpha blockers, 22
alpha tocopherol, 185-186
American Heart Association, 18
    diet, 58-59
anger, 46-47, 137-138
angina pectoris, 14, 20, 37
angioplasty, 2, 15
antibiotics, 198
antidepressants, 198
antioxidants, 19, 41, 182, 184-186
anxiety, 45-46
appetite, 75
    alcohol and, 106
    exercise and, 25
    low-fat diet and, 34
appetizers (recipes), 217-220
arteries, hardening of, 9, 14
ascorbic acid, 184-185
atherosclerosis, 9, 14, 19
    low-fat diet and, 35

baking methods, 69
beans, 72 (table), 73-74
behavior modification, 141-149,
    283-286
beta blockers, 22
beta carotene, 41, 182, 204
    sources, 182 (table)
beverages, 92
biotin, 184
blood pressure, 22
    exercise and, 166, 167
breads (recipes), 221-225
breakfast ideas, 207-208
buckwheat, 93
bulgur, 93
bypass surgery, 2

calciferol, 185
calcium channel blockers, 22
calcium, 41-42
    osteoporosis and, 128-129
    sources, 129 (table)
cancer, 127-128, 130-131,
    201-206
    dietary fat and, 37
    fiber and, 40
    soybeans and, 73

298

capers, 93
carbohydrates, 39-41
cardiovascular medications, 197
catheterization, cardiac, 1-2
chest pain, 14, 20
chick peas, 93
cholesterol, 7, 17-20, 36
    diet and serum, 18
    soybeans and, 73
claudication, 14
colestipol, 6, 7
condiments, 43, 64-67, 71
cooking methods, 64, 69, 76
coronary artery bypass grafting
    (CABG), 15-16
couscous, 93
cross training, 158-162
cyanocobalamin, 184

depression, 47-48
    medications, 198
desserts, 92, 275-281 (recipes)
diabetes, 20, 22-23
diet,
    American Heart Association,
        58-59
    atherosclerosis and, 35
    exercise and, 6
    Healthy Heart Formula,
        59-61
    low-fat, 33-35
    rating of, 53-57
    standard American, 57-58
dietary fat, 17-18, 35, 36 (table),
    37-38
    cancer and, 202-203
    recommended levels, 60-61
dietary supplements, 181-192
dining out, 99-122
diuretics, 22

drugs, 22, 193-199
    antibiotics, 198
    antidepressants, 198
    cardiovascular, 197
    study results and, 6-7

eating out,
    buffets, 115
    cafeteria foods, 113-114
    ethnic foods, 108-113
    foreign language translations,
        118-122
    pizza, 114
    steak houses, 115
eating plan, 59-61, 209-216
    healthy heart, 33
entrées (recipes), 244-269
equipment, exercise, 162-166
estrogen,
    heart disease and, 127, 128
    osteoporosis and, 129, 187
exercise, 24-26, 151-172
    aerobic, 166
    appetite and, 25
    benefits of, 25, 48-50
    blood pressure and, 166, 167
    diet and, 6
    equipment, 151, 162-166
    heart rate and, 158 (table)
    metabolism and, 25
    planning, 155-157
    precautions, 167, 168-170

fat, dietary, 17-18, 33, 35-36
    cancer and, 202-203
    recommended levels, 60-61
fatigue, 47
fiber, dietary, 40-41
    cancer and, 203
    sources, 203 (table)

fitness, 151-172
   cancer and, 204
   rating of, 152
folic acid, neural tube defects
   and, 89
food labels, 82-90
food preparation, 63-73, 74-79
food,
   fast, 99-105
   shopping for, 81-92
   storage of, 95
foreign language translations,
   118-122
fruits, 91

garbanzo beans, 93
genetics, atherosclerosis and, 27
Glucophage, 23
goal setting, 145
grains, 90
group support, 47-48

health claims, product, 84-89
health, predictors of, 5
heart attack, 14
   causes of, 20-21
   incidence of (chart), 14
heart disease,
   men and, 124-125
   risk factors and, 126
   signs of reversal, 10
   women and, 123-132
heart rate, exercise and,
   158, (table)
herbs, 65-67
high blood pressure, 21
hormone supplementation,
   127-130
hypertension, 21

ingredient substitutions, 69

ingredients,
   fat-free, 97
   vegetarian, 93-94
iron, 42

joint problems, exercise and, 25

kasha, 93

labels, food, 82-90
legumes, 91
lentils, 93
lovastatin, 6-7

meal planning, 74-79, 209-216
meat substitutes, 71-73
medications, 22, 193-199
   antibiotics, 198
   antidepressants, 198
   cardiovascular, 197
   study results and, 6-7
meditation, 45
men, heart disease and, 124-125
menopause, 127-130, 187
metabolism, exercise and, 25
metformin, 23
milk, fat content of, 89
millet, 93
minerals, 41-42
miso, 94
motivation, 141-145, 146, 283-286
myocardial infarction, 14, 18

niacin, 6, 183
nicotine, 26-27, 173-179
nicotinic acid, 6
nutrition goals, 52-53
nutrition rating, 53-57
nutritional yeast, 94

oil, sesame, 94
olestra, 98

osteoporosis, 128-129

pancreatitis, 20
pantothenic acid, 183-184
phytochemicals, 189-190, 203-204
pine nuts, 94
pizza, eating out, 114
plaque, arterial, 18
pravastatin, 6, 7
Preventive Health Institute, xvii, 4
produce, organic, 68
products,
  fat-free, 95-98
  low-fat, 95-97
progestin, heart disease and, 127
protein, 33-34, 38, 39 (table)
  sources, 91
  soy, 73
pyridoxine, 184

quinoa, 94

recipe make-overs, 77-79
recipes, 207-281 (see index headings such as appetizers and entrees)
relaxation techniques, 138, 140-141
restaurant food, 99-122
  chain, 115-117
riboflavin, 183
risk factors, heart disease, 9, 17-31, 126

SAD (standard American diet), 57-58
salads, 104-105, 232-238 (recipes)
salt, 42, 67
sandwiches, 70-71
sauces (recipes), 239-243
sea vegetables, 94

seitan, 71
sesame oil, 94
shopping tips, grocery, 81-82, 90-92
side dishes (recipes), 270-274
simvastatin, 7
smoking, 26-27, 173-179
snacks, 75, 92, 149
sodium, 42, 67
soups, 226-231
soy protein, 73
soy sauce, 94
spices, 64-67
steak houses, eating out, 115
stress, 28-31, 43-45, 133-137, 139 (chart)
stretching, 49
stroke, hypertension and, 21
supplements, dietary, 181-192
surgery, types of, 15-16
swimming, 151
Syndrome X, 23

tempeh, 72-73
textured vegetable protein, 72
thiamin, 183
tofu, 71-72
travel, eating out, 118-122
triglycerides, 20-21

vegetables, 90-91
  sea, 94
vegetarian ingredients, 93-94
vitamins, 41, 68, 182-187
  vitamin A, 41
  vitamin A, 182
  vitamin B_1, 183
  vitamin B_2, 183
  vitamin B_3, 183
  vitamin B_5, 183-184
  vitamin B_6, 184
  vitamin B_{12}, 34, 184

vitamin C, 41, 184-185
vitamin D, 185
vitamin E, 19, 41, 185 (table),
    186, 191

walking, 151
water aerobics, 151
water, as a nutrient, 42-43
women,
    heart disease and, 123-132
    stroke and, 124

yeast, nutritional, 94